START LATE, STAY LIGHT

START
LATE
STAY
LIGHT

LIVE A HAPPY, HEALTHY LIFE
WITHOUT GIVING UP THE
FOODS YOU LOVE

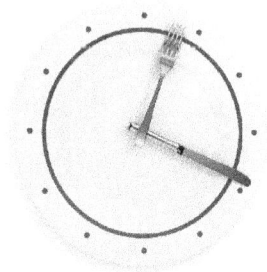

ADAM MARTIN

START LATE, STAY LIGHT

Live a Happy, Healthy Life without
Giving Up the Foods You Love

ISBN   978-1-61961-580-9 *Special Edition*

978-1-61961-578-6 *Paperback*

978-1-61961-579-3 *Ebook*

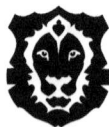

LIONCREST
PUBLISHING

To my amazing wife, Amy, who gives me strength
and courage every day to pursue my dreams
and to never stop believing in myself.

CONTENTS

PREFACE

Congratulations on taking the first step to becoming a later-day eater! Before you dive in, however, I want to briefly tell you what you can expect out of this book.

I've taken more than fifteen years of knowledge, research, and experience within the fitness industry and consolidated it to present a sustainable fitness lifestyle I call Start Late, Stay Light.

Within the pages of this book, you'll learn about how breakfast isn't the most important meal of the day; how calories are broken down into three major macronutrients (what they are, why they're important, and how to calculate your own), and how to incorporate exercise in a way to sustain you for many years to come. Following the content of the book, I've laid out a sixteen-week program (meal plans and training schedules) that anyone can pick up and start—regardless of what level you're starting from or how big your goals are.

More importantly, this book will teach you how to recalibrate what happiness means to you and how doing so will assist you in reaching your health and fitness goals, whatever they may be.

INTRODUCTION

SEVEN DIETS IN SEVEN WEEKS

As an exercise physiologist, I've predominately helped people rebound from injuries, and sometimes that means helping them lose weight. However, the main focus of my career has revolved around exercise and how it can help people live a better life. With my mother's and sister's weight becoming an ever-increasing issue over the past several years, my focus shifted to find an effective weight-loss strategy that would work for them. Family has been (and always will be) the most important aspect of my life, especially after becoming a dad for the first time in 2016.

Despite unloading my entire spiel of knowledge on how to lose weight to my sister and mum, who mean so much to me, nothing seemed to work long-term. Part of the problem is that the "secret" to losing weight is delivered in the same prepackaged cardboard box that the entire industry sends to everyone: "Move more, eat less." The package may come in a variety of shapes and forms—whether that's committing to a paleo or vegetarian diet or joining a CrossFit gym—but it always comes down to eating less and moving more.

Over the last decade or so, I've watched my sister, Sarah, gradually put on weight—and a lot of it. She used to be an active, average-weight teenager, but at the age of thirty, she had gained so much weight that she basically needed to lose about sixty kilos to return to a healthy-weight range. I didn't want to bury my sister at the age of forty, knowing I could have done more to help her. I tried everything under the sun to educate her, encourage her, and try new things with her, but it all ended up being that same prepackaged cardboard-box message, "You should be moving more and eating less."

"Sarah, you should quit sugar. It seems to be the thing that's impeding your health. Stop eating sugar."

"You need to join a gym."

"Sarah, you can't eat pizza. Or ice cream. Or bread."

"You need to start lifting weights."

"Sorry, Sarah. No more desserts."

For the last ten years that I've run my business, I admit I've been guilty of giving my clients the same prepackaged message of "move more, eat less," too. The message rang with some people, and they succeeded in reaching their goals; but others, like my sister, struggled to stick to anything that worked for them long-term. I demonised popular diets, too, telling clients they shouldn't follow programs that restricted carbohydrates, encouraged a higher fat content, or cut out meat. I'd say all these things, yet I had never given any of them a go myself.

Well, shame on me.

A part of me thought maybe there was something to these diets, since a good portion of people often found a benefit to them. I began to think that maybe I shouldn't be too quick to judge these diets, thereby giving my family members and clients the same, prepackaged message of "move more, eat less." Maybe I would discover something in them that could work for Sarah, my mother, and my clients.

Being the accredited exercise physiologist that I am, in

June 2015, I decided to dive headfirst and try seven of the more popular diets out there, one week at a time. I wanted to learn firsthand about these different fad diets and why some people swear by them yet others fail them. More importantly, I started the series in hopes to come across a diet that could work for my sister and my mother (among other clients who struggle with losing weight as well). As I started each week with a new set of rules and regiments, I went *all in*, meaning that instead of easing myself into the diet, I would skip through any "beginning stages" and jump straight into the deep end. I completely committed myself to each program's restrictions from the get-go and made it my goal not to cheat.

For one week at a time, I became a strict vegetarian, a strict paleo, and so on. I did everything to the absolute letter to see how my body would react and how I'd feel, and then I shared my experience via my YouTube channel. On the seventh day of each diet, I sat down in front of my camera and summed up my thoughts, experiences, challenges, successes, and failures. I had a series of questions I asked myself for each week: Was this diet expensive? Was it easy to follow? How did I feel? How did my body react? Was it easy to find produce in that particular program? I was pretty graphic about it as well, when appropriate. I talked about everything, from my surprising bowel movements as a vegetarian to my hatred of sugar-free chocolate cake during my zero-sugar week. Nothing was off the table, and I gave viewers a complete rundown of how they might feel if they tried any of these popular diets.

Which diets did I try? I quit sugar for the first week, became a vegetarian for week two, ate paleo during week three, avoided all gluten for week four, and drank nothing but juice during week five. Week six was the If It Fits Your Macros diet, and for the seventh and final week, I ordered from and ate prepped meals from Lite n' Easy, a commercial-based diet where all the meals are planned out and delivered straight to your door. Here are my takeaways.

WEEK ONE: QUITTING SUGAR

I've never been a big advocate of quitting sugar or subscribed to the idea that sugar is bad for us. If you have some sugar in your diet, it's not the worst thing in the world. Admittedly, people eat far too much of it in our modern diet, and the real problem lies in the huge amounts of additional sugar that are "hidden" in our foods. I definitely recommend reducing the amount of sugar because the amount a typical person consumes these days is too high.

There's a book called *I Quit Sugar* by Sarah Wilson, and it was the book I looked to during my seven-day, sugar-free experiment. Now mind you, she's not a nutritionist, nor is she a health guru. There are a lot of people (celebrities or well-followed fitness people) who write books yet don't have any formal or licensed knowledge in nutrition, health, or fitness—so buyer beware! I encourage you to do your due diligence and check the claims people make before wholly believing in what they're saying (and feel free to check the claims I make in this book, too!).

Wilson starts her eight-week program with baby steps, advising each week to eliminate different obvious sweet and processed foods loaded with sugar until you reach the eighth and final week and have successfully rid your diet of all forms of sugar—from glucose to fructose. I jumped straight to week eight and didn't eat the foods she dictated, meaning I cut out all sugar overnight. Again, since I only dedicated one week to each of these diets, I didn't have the time to "ease into" them.

I should mention I have a ridiculously sensational tooth for sweets. I make sure I eat a little something sweet every day because I know myself, and if I restrict sugar, I'll end up purging on a liter of ice cream at some point. For someone who loves sweet treats, cutting out sugar is purely unrealistic. This is true for me, and I see it within a lot of my clients as well. If I tell someone he or she can no longer have chocolate (or whatever this person's favourite sweet thing in the world is), I know that within three or four weeks time, this person will binge on it and (of course) not tell me. When it's time to check in and he or she is not showing any results, the inevitable question comes out: "Have you cheated this week?"

"No, no. I didn't eat chocolate this week."

"That's not what the scale says..."

Let's face it, not eating the things we love is miserable, and the bottom line is that it's not sustainable.

I think most people on the planet love sugar. It's what our brain craves, and it's in our genetics, stemming from our hunter-gatherer days. I hate using that terminology, but it's true. Back then, not having readily available food on a shelf, the brains of our Paleolithic brothers and sisters craved sweet things because they were energy. They ate berries to satisfy those cravings, and we still have that ingrained need for sweetness from sugar because it means survival.

You might hear from time to time that our brain reacts to sugar similarly to the way it reacts to amphetamines. Your brain definitely has a hormonal response that says eating sugar is good. No matter who you are, there's not a person on this planet who doesn't like sweet things in some way, shape, or form. For someone, it might be lollies. For someone else, it might be chocolate. For others still, it might be fruit. Regardless, sweet things are good for us.

I didn't cheat in the "Quitting Sugar" week, but by the end of the week, my sweet tooth was uncontrollable, and I was dying for something sweet and tasty, even if it was some fruit. I missed being able to eat a banana, for example. A diet without bananas? Come on!

The downfall of this diet and why I don't think it works is that it's simply not sustainable.

WEEK TWO: VEGETARIAN

Eating vegetarian for a week was full of surprises. First of all, I'm a carnivore. I love my meat, and I'm a big advocate of people eating more protein (because people typically don't include enough protein in their diet), so heading into the vegetarian week did not excite me in the slightest. You can certainly get protein through vegetarian sources like soybeans, tofu, and falafel, for example, but I enjoy eating protein much more when it comes from an animal.

I thought I would struggle not eating meat, but I quite enjoyed it. It forced me to explore outside my usual comfort zone of animal products, resulting in a considerable change in flavours. I came across some great recipes, and they were all surprisingly delicious. Without getting too graphic, my bowel movements massively changed—and I'm a pretty regular-type guy—but I was on the toilet quite a bit since I ate more vegetables and fibre. I tend to eat quite a lot of vegetables in my normal diet as is, but even so, it was a noticeable change, and I was quite surprised at how quickly it happened.

In my YouTube review, I said it would behoove us all to dedicate at least one day a week to eating vegetarian. For those who are physically active, it won't hinder your performance or your movement; however, it might be wise to time your meat-free day on a rest day. If you were planning for a heavy weight-training session, I would eat meat on that day. In general, though, I think it would be a good idea if all of us added a meat-free day to our weekly plan. You can think of it like a rest a day, but for your mouth and gut.

Going vegetarian for a week also saved me a heap of money. Protein is expensive, so not buying steak, chicken, and fish for the week meant more money in my pocket. In that week alone, I saved sixty to seventy dollars by not buying meat.

WEEK THREE: PALEO

I probably shouldn't have staged it this way, but I went

from vegetarian in one week to paleo the next, which is basically an all-meat diet. Needless to say, my body received quite the shock come Monday morning when I started eating paleo. This program certainly has its advocates, and people are either for it or dead against it.

If you enjoy meat, you'll love paleo; but if you love grains, you'll hate paleo.

There is definitely something to the philosophy behind it, and while there's been a few celebrities who advocate the paleo diet (again, be sure to check your sources!), it's still not sustainable, especially for those who enjoy pasta, bread, and cereals.

Overall, I enjoyed eating paleo because I'm a carnivore and I never went hungry, but not eating grains was a definite challenge.

Surprisingly, some research suggests the reason why we developed as a species is not because we started eating meat but because we started eating grains and other starchy carbs, giving the brain the required energy it needs to function day to day.[1] Grains, breads, cereals, and quite a lot of different vegetables that are prohibited from the

1   "Starchy Carbs, Not Paleo, Advanced the Human Race," University of Sydney, August 10, 2015, http://sydney.edu.au/news-opinion/news/2015/08/10/starchy-carbs--not-a-paleo-diet--advanced-the-human-race.html

paleo diet are excellent energy sources, and I don't understand the rationale behind why they're not allowed.

Of course, the typical responses from die-hard paleos are, "Well, the caveman didn't have it back then, so we shouldn't have it now; the reason we're all unhealthy is because we're eating bread."

Um, no.

Advocates love to argue that cavemen lived healthier lives, so we should therefore eat like them. Excuse me? The average life span of a caveman was twenty-five years, whereas the average lifespan now is eighty—who is really living better lives? I'm pretty sure we are. The rationale behind it doesn't make sense to me. Granted, I know advances in medicine have played a significant part in our longevity, but to say bread, pasta, and potatoes are behind our unhealthier modern lives, in my opinion, is plain ridiculous.

Regardless of rationales and explanations, the paleo diet, although one that didn't make me go hungry, is still too restrictive, and I don't find that sustainable.

WEEK FOUR: GLUTEN-FREE

Not only did I avoid eating gluten for this week, but I also made it a point to try all the gluten-free products people buy instead of eating the gluten equivalent. I bought gluten-free pasta, gluten-free bread, gluten-free chips, and a bunch of other kinds of gluten-free products sold on grocery shelves everywhere.

In my opinion, the gluten-free craze is a big fad that's been pushed by—shocker—celebrities, fitness gurus, and some health professionals claiming gluten is the devil and the reason why people are unhealthy.

Sigh.

There is extremely little evidence to suggest eating gluten is of any detriment to your health whatsoever—unless you have a medical condition like coeliac disease. It's estimated that 1 to 1.5 percent of the population have coeliac disease, and they 100 percent can't eat gluten because it's going to kill them or make them terribly ill. Then there's about 4 to 8 percent of the population (depending on the kind of data you pull up) who have some sort of intolerance, but not to a degree that would kill them. What happens if these people ate some gluten? They might feel a bit bloated.

In all honesty, the gluten-free week was a bit of a joke to me, and there was no way you could ever convince me gluten is bad for you. I have no problem—and will never have a problem—with people eating bread. Obviously you can't eat twenty slices of bread for lunch and expect it to have a positive result. However, bread, cereals, and pasta—like everything else—is good in moderation. It's not the gluten in these products that's making people unhealthy; it's that they're eating an entire loaf of bread as opposed to two slices.

My heart goes out to those with coeliac disease because I probably would jump off a bridge if I was ever diagnosed. I'd finish my life early because I don't want to live a life without bread or pasta.

Bottom line: Don't worry about going gluten-free unless you have to for health-related reasons. Period.

WEEK FIVE: JUICE CLEANSE

Whenever I hear the phrase "juice cleanse," I picture someone like Gwyneth Paltrow promoting her so-called holistic elimination diet, juicing some exotic berries found in the depths of the Himalayas.

Excuse me while I roll my eyes.

First of all, this is not a diet. A juice cleanse—sometimes also referred to as a detox—is the furthest thing away from being sustainable, not only compared to the other diets in my experiment, but also compared to *any* other diet out there.

I came across Joe Cross, and I watched on Netflix his movie that came out in 2010, *Fat, Sick, and Nearly Dead*. He was an overweight, forty-year-old executive who had a heart issue, and this documentary followed him when he went on this big, "I'm going to juice everything in my life" journey to lose weight and get healthy. He juice-fasted for ninety days, shed an amazing amount of kilos, and turned his life around. If you look him up today, he's kept most of the weight off and lives a healthy, balanced life.

I remember thinking, *Well, okay. Maybe I shouldn't roll my eyes at this. Let's say there's something to it. This guy seemed to change and turn his life around. Why couldn't other people do it? Let's have a go.*

Heading into this juicing week, because my calorie intake would be so low, I had to limit my exercise (boo). I bought Cross's smartphone app and made some of the juice recipes found there, which I'll admit were pretty interesting. The juices were flavoursome and different than some of the juices I've had before, but I'm not a big advocate of drinking calories; I'd rather eat them.

I survived through day one relatively easily. On day two, I started getting grumpy, and by day three, I was ready to murder someone.

I really, really struggled. Cross warns newbies about some of the early struggles (headache, lethargic, lack of focus), and in his documentary, he explains that days three, four, and five are the toughest, and once you survive them, things get easier.

By day three, I became snappy at my family and my clients due to my hunger, at which point my wife said, "You have to eat something because you're becoming unbearable." I was ravenous and had no energy. I needed fuel, and the juices weren't enough. Drinking juices day in and day out was miserable. I missed eating. I missed chewing things. When I made it to day four, I had a workout planned and almost passed out. I became really light-headed and starry eyed, and that's when I decided to pull the plug.

It was the only diet out of the seven that I quit.

Oh!—and it's not like I grabbed a salad or a banana when I quit. Oh no, no, no, no. I drove to the store and bought a tub of ice cream, ate it all, and then ate a whole loaf of bread afterward! I went off the deep end.

But you know what? I instantly felt better.

After gorging myself on some not-so-healthy options (but so delicious!), I did finish the rest of the week off juicing. There is no chance I would ever juice for a full thirty days, let alone do what Joe Cross did in his documentary and juice for ninety—no way. There might be a small percent of the population who can hold out for thirty days, and I'd be the first to shake their hands and congratulate them—good on you! If this is the start you need to lose some weight and get going, full power to you, but juicing certainly was never going to work for me.

I calculated (for fun—oh yeah, I'm a real party animal!) how much food I would need to reach my daily calorie intake, which is usually around 2,000 to 2,200 calories, give or take (depending on the day). I would have to juice a ridiculous amount of food in order to reach a calorie level to sustain me. I would wear out several Magic Bullets trying to juice that amount of food every day, and I'd destroy juicers on a weekly basis!

I drank between 450 and 800 calories a day, depending on if I used nut-based juices or vegetable- or fruit-based juices. Even on an inactive day, my baseline is probably 1,600 to 1,800 calories, which meant I was missing out on a minimum of 1,000 calories a day. If I did this for thirty days, I would have been a skeleton by the end of it.

Juicing is not a diet and will never be something sustainable long-term. You may be able to get away with it for a few weeks and drop some weight, and if it's what you need to build some momentum to begin your weight-loss journey, then I say go for it. That is where it should stop, though, as this is not a long-term option.

WEEK SIX: IF IT FITS YOUR MACROS

If It Fits Your Macros, or IIFYM, is quite popular in the body-building scene but has made its way into the mainstream thanks to fitness professionals using social media—go search the hashtag "IIFYM" to see how many posts exist in Instagram. In a broad nutshell, you can basically eat what you like as long as it fits your macros. It doesn't matter if you eat fruit loops or if you eat a potato—a carbohydrate is a carbohydrate. It doesn't matter if fat is monounsaturated or polyunsaturated because a fat is a fat. A protein is a protein whether you get that from a protein shake or a steak.

What is a macro? Macro is the shortened word for

macronutrient, which is what makes up our food. There are three major macros: protein, carbohydrates, and fats. Alcohol is also considered a macro, but that is a story for another day. The calories associated with macronutrients are the calories that make up our food. One gram of protein has four calories, one gram of carbohydrate also has four calories, and one gram of fat has nine calories. In case you were wondering, alcohol has seven calories per gram. When I dial out a client's plan, I break down how many macronutrients he or she needs to eat for his or her specific body type and goals. For example, one client could need 150 grams of protein a day, 100 grams of carbohydrates, and 35 grams of fat. That breakdown equals a certain amount of calories that this client would strive to eat each day.

When I first learned about IIFYM, it instantly intrigued me. I searched to see if anyone in my sphere followed this plan and found a colleague at work who did. He strictly follows a IIFYM lifestyle and has a phenomenal body (he's competed in body-building competitions both locally and internationally). I remember thinking that there must be something to this IIFYM since he's found it quite beneficial to himself *and* promotes it to all his clients.

I figured out my macros based off of several factors (we'll get into this later in the book), and I planned my week of workouts and meals, which happened to include ice cream. I asked the guy at work, who has followed IIFYM religiously for about two years, if he could look over my plan. He did and gave me his stamp of approval, and I was ecstatic. How cool was this? I could eat green veggies and some chicken for lunch, a burger for dinner, and then enjoy some ice cream for dessert.

I started researching some more, and through a Google search, I came across a guy named Mike Vacanti. Mike is also a big advocate of tracking your macros, sporting an outrageous body that even my wife claims is the best she's ever seen. A lot of what Mike and my work colleague talked about not only made sense to me, but seemed simple to follow if you were willing to do a little work.

Overall, I found the IIFYM diet to be of great benefit. The only flaw I saw in it was that it is extremely pedantic. Its biggest downside is people won't be prepared to put in the work. It is quite difficult to track all your food, knowing exactly what you're putting in your mouth and how many macros are in each item, and it takes an enormous amount of time, mostly in the beginning. A lot of people three or four weeks in say, "You know what? I'm done with this. It's too difficult to measure and count every little bit of food I'm eating, and I'm fed up."

WEEK SEVEN: LITE N' EASY

Lite n' Easy is a weight-loss company that delivers prepped meals straight to your door. Since they only deliver once a week, you make your meal choices on their website in advance, depending on what program you choose. Lite n' Easy offers three programs: a 1,800 calorie meal plan, a 1,500 calorie meal plan, or a 1,200 calorie plan. The website walks you through a series of questions, and then an entire week of meals is mapped out for you. You don't have to do anything whatsoever in terms of cooking or preparing, but it's not cheap. I'd argue, however, that if you think about the eating habits of most people, they're probably spending about the same as they usually would, if they added up all the coffee runs and lunch dates they go on during a typical workweek. If you're someone who makes your own meals for lunch and dinner, though, then it's definitely more expensive.

The meals are delivered with a schedule of what you should eat on which day and when. All you have to do is pick your day one and follow what the program tells you to eat for breakfast, lunch, and dinner. It's simple and super convenient.

To my surprise, by the end my one-week experiment, I was a big advocate. Lite n' Easy is a fantastic way of introducing people to weight loss because they'll see exactly what appropriate portions look like. Most people say, "Yeah, I eat healthy. I eat steak and veggies for dinner, and I have a sandwich for lunch," but the steak they eat is a four-hundred-gram piece of steak coupled with a mountain of mashed potatoes.

Sure, they're eating so-called "clean" foods, but they're eating too much of them. While the portions from Lite n' Easy might seem small, we've grown accustomed to huge overflowing plates and eating everything on them. Lite n' Easy's portions aren't small portions; they are correct portions, which I found to be this week's number-one benefit.

The food wasn't that bad, either. I thought these pre-packaged meals would be heavily salted to cover up the blandness and be full of unhealthy hidden ingredients. I thought they would taste like plastic, but all the food throughout the day was fresh. There were sandwiches, salads, fruits, and muesli. All the dinners took seven minutes in the microwave, but again, to be honest, they weren't that bad; they were quite flavoursome.

Despite the cost, I think services like Lite n' Easy are hugely beneficial to people who struggle with weight loss. It's convenient, it's easy, and if you stick to it, you'll definitely lose some weight. The problem is the price tag, which isn't sustainable for those on a budget.

NOW YOU TRY

The Seven Diets in Seven Weeks series was a hugely beneficial experiment, and I'm glad I did it. I encourage you also to give it a go. Before you start my program, dedicate a week of your life to each of these fad diets (or try others that I didn't), and take note of how your body reacts. It's an amazing experiment to try on yourself, and I promise you will learn a ton. If you haven't done so already, I want you to exhaust through every diet out there before trying mine out.

The seven diets I tried fall into the same category as all the other fad diets we've seen come and go over the years: they're not lifestyles that are sustainable. Sure, you can follow any program for ten weeks and lose some weight, but once the program is over, you'll revert to your old habits and gain back the weight you've lost, and probably then some. Sadly, this is exactly what 98 percent of the population ends up doing, regardless of the diet or program.

I remember thinking, *There has to be something different out there—something that would work for my sister and my mum.*

I'm a YouTube fanboy and use it as a search engine for everything—from learning how to change a LED light bulb to repairing a puncture in a bike tire. When I first stumbled upon If It Fits Your Macros, I didn't know what that meant, so off to YouTube I went. When looking further into IIFYM, I also came across the term "intermittent fasting." Intermittent fasting is a pattern of eating and is a way of scheduling your meals so you get the most out of them. Intermittent fasting doesn't change *what* you eat; it changes *when* you eat.

The first YouTube video I came across while diving into intermittent fasting was of a guy named Greg O'Gallagher. He is the creator of Kinobody, a workout program focusing on intermittent fasting (and mostly marketed to men seeking to improve their physical bodies to attract women). When I stumbled upon Greg—who didn't eat in the morning and had a physique like a general in a Spartan army—I thought maybe there was something more to skipping breakfast that I wasn't aware of, so I started to dig a little deeper. We've all heard those popular sayings about the importance of eating in the morning—many of which I admit I have repeated to my own clients. These sayings include "Eat like a king in the morning and eat like the poor at night" and "You should have your most important meal at the start of the day." Yet here was this guy, Greg, who skipped breakfast and sported an incredibly built and strong physique. Clearly, omitting calories at the start of his day didn't deter him from making gains and maintaining health.

I dove back into the Interwebs to research more and not base my opinions solely on a fit-looking guy who was mostly concerned about his looks and helping guys pick up girls with their amazing biceps. I looked for published studies about fasting to see if it was truly beneficial for your body or if Greg was a phoney, marketing his products to make money. Greg's philosophy and marketing come from what I call a "bro science" kind of place—which is fine, I guess, if you're into that sort of thing. What I mean is that he sells his products with messages like "how to pick up girls" or "how to look good for women" or "how to lift heavier in the gym so the ladies will want to touch you." Well, that's fine for maybe 5 percent of the male population (maybe more if males were truly honest about why they go to the gym) who are motivated by such factors, but it's not the demographic I'm trying to target, and it most certainly is not the category my sister and mother fall into.

I looked at the science behind fasting in general, and in researching, I stumbled upon another diet that involved fasting: the 5:2 diet, otherwise known as the Fast Diet, founded by Mike Mosley, a doctor in the UK. The basic concept behind the Fast Diet, as discussed in Mosley's book *The Fast Diet*, is to eat normally for five days a week and then to eat highly restricted calories on the other two days; the restricted days, or the fasting days, do not have to be consecutive days.

I didn't try the 5:2; I didn't need to because I know myself, especially after what happened during the juice cleanse. If I were restricted to no more than 500 calories on any day, it would make me miserable. I consider myself a pretty average guy, so I'm guessing that the majority of others wouldn't succeed with this, either. More importantly, my mum and sister trying to fast for an entire day or two per week was never something they would do long-term.

I appreciated the 5:2 diet because scientific data backed its claims. That the founder is a doctor gave me the validation I was looking for as well. When Dr. Mosley was in his early fifties, he was diagnosed with diabetes. His father, who passed away from heart failure at the age of seventy-four, was also diagnosed with diabetes. Fearing a similar fate, Dr. Mosley heard about possible links between fasting and how it can benefit your health, not only for those who wish to lose weight, but also for those with type 2 diabetes, hypertension, cardiovascular risk, Alzheimer's, dementia, and Parkinson's disease. Rather than start on medication, he started researching and experimenting, subsequently leading him to the 5:2 diet, by which he lost ten kilos and successfully reversed his diabetes. In addition, other health markers, such as cholesterol and blood pressure, improved. What's even more amazing is that both his weight and his blood sugars have remained normal ever since.

My nan passed away from Parkinson's and Alzheimer's, so I thought maybe there was something to this intermittent fasting that could help people. I loved Dr. Mosley's science behind fasting and how it could help with health and longevity. He was successful in popularising it because he's a doctor (so he's highly respected) and since he's done a lot of health and wellness documentaries, too, including one on the Fast Diet. I respect him because he's an experimental doctor, meaning he loves experimenting rather than reading something and pushing it onto his patients. I see myself in him in a way because he offers himself as a guinea pig to research and only advocates things that have personally worked for him, which is exactly what I do (even though I am no doctor).

There's also research on those who fast during Ramadan; they fast for the entire day, and their health seems to get better during this period. Research says calorie restriction is a stress for our bodies, and experiencing stresses is a good thing—not a bad thing. We live in a world where food is readily available, and we don't truly experience stress, except for perceived stress. I don't want to gloss over stress in people's lives, but I think we perceive certain things and situations to be much more stressful than they really are.

What I mean by stresses on our bodies is physical stresses,

such as when you go without food for an extended period of time, and your body has a stress response to it. It stems back to our early caveman days with our instinctual fight-or-flight response. When your body knows it's hungry, it thinks, "My reactions need to become better because I need to be able to find food or else I'm going to die." That kind of response doesn't naturally happen in us anymore, because when we're hungry, we simply walk over to the cupboard and grab something to put in our mouth. The body therefore never undergoes stress over survival, and it never ignites the fight-or-flight response.

Your body has about fourteen to sixteen hours worth of glycogen in your muscles and your liver, so once that's tapped up after a long fasting period, your body says, "Now what? I need to find energy from somewhere else." That's when your body begins tipping into your fat stores and your growth hormones start to go up. Most people think, *If I don't have breakfast, I'll feel lethargic and low.* You might feel that for the first two days because you've conditioned your body to expect food in the morning, but that's normal in any new regimen—your body needs time to adjust.

Basically, we can manufacture the fight-or-flight response because it's in our DNA.

When your body is digesting, it needs energy to digest your food, so it can't perform other functions. That's why we've always been told to avoid swimming right after eating a meal, because you're more likely to experience tummy cramps. When you eat food, your body pushes blood toward your stomach to digest the food, which means there's less blood circulating in your extremities, making it dangerous to go swimming. If you don't have food in your system and you don't have any thing circulating around your body, your body can perform other functions. If your body isn't digesting, its energy diverts and goes to other areas where it can be it more useful.

There's even some early, early research that's suggesting that this rejuvenation of cells in the body while it's fasting is good for your skin, making you look better (hello, fountain of youth!).

All of this research supports Dr. Mosley's 5:2 diet of eating whatever you'd like for five days and then fasting for the remaining two. I knew fasting for two days was never going to work for me long-term, so I wanted to see if skipping breakfast or prolonging a fast would result in the same health benefits that a full day of fasting did.

Turns out, a sixteen-hour fast seems to have surprisingly similar benefits to the 5:2 diet.

People often think fasting is bad for you, but they fail to realise we already do it: We all fast when we sleep. Let's say you go to bed at 10:00 p.m., and your last meal was at 8:00 p.m., and you don't eat again until 8:00 the next morning. You've fasted for twelve hours! Everyone fasts for about ten to twelve hours every night as it is, so if you prolong that fast for another four hours, you'll get the same benefits as if you fasted an entire day.

ENTER LATER-DAY EATING

When I first started skipping breakfast, I knew right away that it would work well for me because I don't typically wake up hungry (I wake up at 4:30 a.m. every day), so I was excited to no longer force myself to eat food in the morning. I'm also a bit OCD in nature and like to know exactly what's happening and when it's happening. I plan out my meals for the week in a smartphone app called MyFitnessPal (which I highly recommend everyone start using). Skipping breakfast was easy, I felt great, and so the early stages of my later-day lifestyle started developing.

It's important to note why I want you to go exhaust your way through every other diet out there. I want Start Late, Stay Light to be your "last first kiss," meaning it will be the last "diet" you'll ever need to try because it'll become not only a lifestyle you'll enjoy, but one that will help you achieve health and happiness. Once you witness for yourself the effectiveness of this program, you'll become a lifelong advocate. The beauty of later-day eating is you can still follow any diet restrictions or diet plans you want. You can make later-day eating a lifestyle if you're a vegetarian or a paleo. All I'm suggesting is you change "when" you start eating. With Start Late, Stay Light, I don't care what diet you follow as long as you don't start eating until around 1:00 in the afternoon.

Tracking your food is immensely important, and I highly recommend that you spend some time practising (start today!); learning what is in your food will pay dividends in the long run. As a starting point, I have mapped out a meal plan for a sixteen-week program (which you can find in the back of this book), but tracking what you eat every day will teach you how many calories and macronutrients your favourite foods contain; it will expose your eating habits—good or bad.

Most of us think we eat a wide variety of foods and that our diets are rich and complex, but in reality, if you track your food, you'll realise you probably only eat six or seven different dinners and two or three different lunches. We tend to eat a lot of the same stuff, especially if they're satisfying and easy to make. Yet somehow, we have this grandiose idea that we eat so many different meals and that we would never be able to remember the macros to all of them. You don't. Once you know the items in the meals you tend to repeat, you can easily work out what you can eat for lunch and dinner to make sure it fits your macros for the day—it just takes time. With enough practise, you'll come to learn about food in a way where you won't have to track every day.

Think of eating calories and counting your macros like a budget. Most people understand the concept of money in, money out, but they somehow don't understand food in, food out. If you earn $1,000 a week and you spend it all on Monday, you won't have any money to spend for the rest of the week. Your diet is exactly the same. If you are given 1,400 calories at the start of the day and eat all of them for breakfast, that means you can't eat anything else for the rest of the day.

Most people inherently don't want to give up their favourite foods, especially at dinner, after dinner, or during social events—all of which are typically consumed toward the end of the day. The best way to continue to indulge in your favourite dinners and desserts is to eliminate breakfast—it's not as important as we thought anyway!—thereby saving calories to enjoy those indulges later in the day.

IIFYM is all about tracking, which forces you to think about your calorie budget for the day, every day. If you have a $1,000 budget for the week, instead of spending it on five little things, you can save and spend the entire $1,000 on one big thing. Similarly, if you're allotted 1,400 calories for the day, and you spread those calories over two meals instead of six, it means those two meals can be bigger—meaning more calories.

Most people don't find fasting until 1:00 in the afternoon too difficult. The real challenge is taking the time to track your food and prioritising mastering this skill over watching the latest episode of *Game of Thrones* or having a beer with friends. I'm not going to sugarcoat this for you, either: Tracking is challenging. It's tedious and time-consuming, but if you stick with it over time, I promise you it will become second nature. I can look at most meals now and guess fairly accurately what macros are in them, which sort of makes me feel like Neo from the first *Matrix* movie, when he finally fully grasps the illusion of the Matrix and sees the green code of ones and zeros. With enough practise—and I mean months, not a few weeks—you can also be the Neo of tracking macros.

It takes time, and everyone—and I mean *everyone*—struggles in the beginning, especially those who have never thought about the macros in their food before. You might be surprised in what you discover. For example, did you know that a McDonald's medium Big Mac meal with fries and a coke (not a diet coke) has less calories than a foot-long tuna sandwich from Subway on its own (with no cheese or dressing, I might add)? It's true!

Foot-long tuna sandwich from Subway with no cheese or dressing:
Calories: 960
Protein: 40g
Carbs: 88g
Fat: 50g

A Big Mac from McDonald's with medium fries:
Calories: 860
Protein: 30g
Carbs: 91g
Fat: 43g

Tracking your food is an essential part of my program, but more so, it's something I think we all should do regardless of our goals, because we don't learn about what is in our food otherwise.

A BIT OF BACKGROUND

I've been active my whole life. I played in a number of different fields, but tennis was my main sport. Unfortunately, a serious injury forced me to give up playing my beloved tennis. While rehabilitating my shoulder, I worked with an exercise physiologist and became fascinated with the field. He was forthcoming and answered all my questions regarding the career, but most of all, I was attracted to his passion for helping others. I decided right then and there to pursue a career in physiology, primarily because I wanted to help people live happier and healthier lives.

I completed a five-year master's degree and did a research project for a hospital in Australia, where I found a niche in the market of people who were coming out of the hospital system. If you were involved in a car collision or a major accident at work, you probably received good in-house services at the hospital and were well taken care of during that period. Once the hospital discharged you, however, you didn't get to take your exercise physiologist home with you to continue your physical therapy and rehabilitation. The hospital would let you go, and say, "Here's your program. Go to your local gym and continue the exercises on your own. Good luck. We wish you well on your journey."

That didn't seem right to me. I remember thinking to myself: *Shouldn't we be doing more for these people before they go hire a personal trainer who has no idea of their injuries that implicate how they need to get back to full fitness?* This small gap in the market was the reason I launched my business, TrewExPhys. I started by working with hospitals, physiotherapists, general practitioners, doctors, and surgeons, and I told them, "Once you're finished with your patient, don't send them to a personal trainer who helps people lose weight; send them to me." And they did. The business has evolved over the past ten years, but I primarily help people return to their lives and enjoy the things they did *before* their injury.

Losing weight was a common goal among many of my clients in helping them reach their rehabilitation goals, but I didn't look deeper into the weight-loss field until I started worrying about my sister's health.

SARAH'S TURN

When I came across the benefits of fasting into lunchtime, I knew I had to try it with Sarah. I was able to convince her slowly that breakfast isn't the most important meal of the day (more on this later). Skipping breakfast didn't restrict her from the foods she loved, either. It was a slow and steady progression, but after the first five weeks, she started losing weight. My sister, who is the most stubborn person when it comes to weight loss, never called to complain and tell me how difficult she was finding it and that she wanted to stop; she kept going.

Ten weeks in, she was down twelve kilos.

My mum picked it up as well and joined my sister. She didn't need to lose as much as Sarah, but carrying around extra weight in your later years can impose various challenges. My mum probably needed to lose twenty kilos, and within the first twenty weeks on the program, she had lost sixteen.

Here's a message I received from my mum:

Hi Gorgeous,

I wanted to say a big THANK YOU to you for all the time, effort, and money you spent over the years in trying to get Sarah and me healthy and lose some weight. Without you, I would not weigh and feel as healthy as I do today. Start Late, Stay Light is something I find easy to do and can also follow and keep up for a lifetime. I am so grateful to you for changing my life for the better. I have a new lease on life, and because of the weight loss, feeling better, and being full of energy, it has also helped with my bad knee. It does not hurt as much, and I can walk further without pain; therefore I exercise more and so lose more weight. In my wildest dreams I would never have thought I could get my weight down into the seventy kilos again. Thank you, thank you from the bottom of my heart. I owe you for giving me my life back.

Love always,
Mum

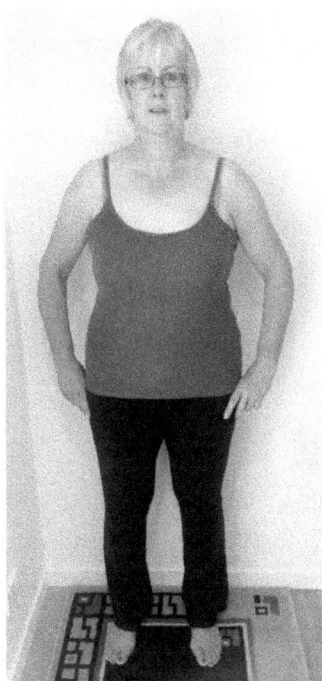

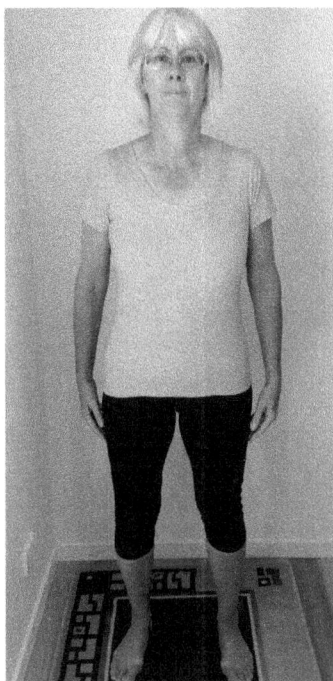

My mum sent that message to me randomly one day, and of course it made my day. She's had knee issues for quite some time and always thought it came with age, but now that she's sixteen kilos lighter, her knee isn't a problem anymore.

Ten months into her journey, Sarah lost thirty-two kilos— which is a phenomenal effort, but she still has a long way to go. When you plug in some numbers, she should be about sixty to sixty-five kilos. She's still working to lose another twenty to twenty-five kilos, so her journey is far from over, whereas my mum reached her goal and has lost a total of twenty-two kilos in the same six-month time frame. Even though my mother reached her weight goal and my sister continues on the path to reaching hers, the journey continues for both of them in maintaining weight. Fitness is a never-ending commitment, and the later-day eating lifestyle will continue to help them for many years to come.

FITNESS ISN'T JUST FOR ABS

I ask all my new clients the same questions: "Why are you here? What are you doing here now? What can I do for you to help you into the future?" The answers I usually hear are these: "You need to fix my knee so I can play sports again," or, "Can you help me with my back problems?" or, "I need to lose weight because I want to find a husband."

A new client came to discuss her goals with me one day, and I will never forget her. She was seventy-five years of age, and her husband had passed away five weeks prior. This lovely lady's response to one of my questions was one I'd never heard before, and it fundamentally changed the way I looked at health, wellness, and fitness (and why it should be important to all of us). She said, "My husband of forty-five years passed away five weeks ago, and my number-one fear is that I'll fall over at home and won't be able to get up to call for help."

I started crying, and then she started crying, and I thought, *Oh, my god; fitness isn't just for abs.* It was a powerful moment for me, and it made me think of my mum's text message saying I'd given her life back in her sixties.

This client's motivation was surely powerful, but all motivation is important—no motivation is superior to another. Although looking good is a great motivator—and I'm the first to admit that I love doing biceps curls and posting topless shots on my Snapchat—more importantly, fitness and taking care of your health through my program will help you live longer so you can spend more time with your loved ones, doing the things you love. We only have one life, and time is a precious commodity; we all want to spend as much time living on this planet with the ones we love and doing the things we love. We can't do that without good health, and good health starts with what we put into our bodies.

YOU'LL HAVE TO WORK FOR IT

"Stop eating breakfast, and all of your worries are done."

I mistakenly said those words in the very, very beginning because the concept was that easy for me. I'm not, however, an overweight person. I do struggle with portion control (like most people), and eating a little too much ice cream happens from time to time, but skipping breakfast was a good way for me to still enjoy my ice cream obsession after dinner, occasional drinks with friends, and my favourite foods. I don't eat too much above and beyond what I should, and most of my exercise keeps me within my limit, so I took my idea of eliminating breakfast and simply told the world, "If you stop eating in the morning, you will lose weight and look fantastic!"

The problem was, I made it sound far too simple. A lot of people who started the program then overcompensated: "Since I'm not eating breakfast, that means I can have twice as much for dinner."

Um, no. That's now how it works.

This lifestyle is not an elixir. When you get into the nuts and bolts of it, there's some hard work to do, and it will take dedication, commitment, and perseverance—which we'll get to in later chapters. The concept is simple, but the actions are not. It is a simple plan to follow—and if you follow it, you will lose weight, you will feel better, and you will get healthier—but by no means is it an easy process to become a later-day eater. It takes practise, like anything else in life worth striving for.

I had to implement more guidelines and more rules to

keep clients in check. Just because you're skipping breakfast doesn't mean you get to sit there and "make up" for it later.

The beauty of this program is you can start this lifestyle tomorrow. You don't have to buy anything special, nor do you have to change anything drastically. You can still eat breakfast foods if you want, too. If you have a box of cereal sitting in your cupboard, don't throw it out; eat it after 1:00 p.m. Despite the time it takes to track food, I don't think it's difficult for anyone to give it a go, either.

In fact, the most difficult part for most people is convincing them breakfast isn't important.

The success rates of diets in the market that offer twelve-week programs are pretty high, believe it or not. Participants lose weight in these twelve-week programs, but when you look at that person two years later, the long-term success rate drops because the majority of the participants regain the weight they lost or, in most cases, put on even more weight. Interestingly, the success rate on my program follows an opposite pattern. As an example, let's say ten people join my program. As the program progresses (and gets more challenging), five people drop out. My success rate for people sticking to the program is therefore 50 percent, which sounds bad, but wait. The kicker is that those five who continue with the program long-term all succeed in reaching their goals, so therefore, my program has a 100 percent success rate for those who stick to it and make it a lifestyle.

We as humans fundamentally do not like change, and that's why I think the later-day lifestyle works best because it disrupts your life as minimally as possible. Take the electric car, for example. We all know they're better for the environment and that we should be driving them, but owning and operating one disrupts our lives far too much. If I wanted to travel one thousand kilometers, I'd only be able to travel a quarter of the way to my destination before I would need to find a place to plug in my car, and I would even need to stay somewhere overnight so the car would have enough time to fully recharge, extending my journey another day. With a car that takes petrol, as soon as it runs low, I simply fill it up at any gas station and keep on driving.

It's exactly the same in the weight-loss world. Too many of these diets try to change you fundamentally. If you're someone who loves sugar, and I tell you, "This diet says you can't have sugar," you'll probably stick it out and not eat sugar for twelve weeks (I certainly wouldn't last that long—I'd quit after a week!), but at some point, that little voice inside your head is going to say, "You want that chocolate bar, don't you?" You can't say no to that forever. And we don't fall off the bandwagon with one chocolate bar, either; we tend to fall off in a big way—like me eating an entire liter of ice cream and an entire loaf of bread after four days of juicing.

You should be able to eat the foods you enjoy, and with later-day eating, you can. In this book, I will teach you how you can still eat that chocolate bar, ice cream, bread, or pasta, as well as enjoy that glass of wine when you're out with friends. I will teach you how to build your favourite foods into this lifestyle. You've read this far (thank you!), and from here on out, I will outline the steps you need to work on to ensure you are successful in living a happier, healthier, and longer life.

It starts by not eating breakfast.

1

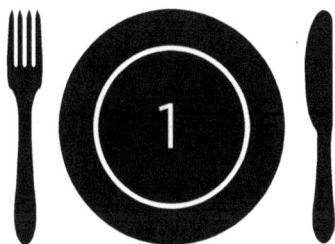

HAPPINESS COMES FIRST

As far back as I can remember, my goal has always been to help one million people live a happier, healthier, and longer life. Seriously—I want to help one million people change their lives.

I've also always wanted to own my dream car, a Lamborghini, and my wife said I could buy one if I sold one million copies of this book—talk about motivation!

In any journey to achieve lofty goals, it's vital to establish your "why."

Why do I wake up at 4:30 a.m. every morning? Why am I

publishing a book? Why am I taking hours out of each day to provide free content to the world on health, wellness, and nutrition? Why do I work out and keep strict(ish) with my food, 95 percent of the time? Why do I push people on my program to keep moving forward?

The answer: To always be the best damn role model for my daughter (and future kids), and to leave a legacy of making a difference in the world so my kids can stand proud to say that it was their dad who did that.

And secondly, to own a Lamborghini (I'm serious—I want one so bad!).

When times are tough and all I want to do is quit and throw in the towel, I think of my "why," and it reminds me to keep going. Find the "why" in you that makes you feel guilty when you aren't giving it your all. Find the "why" within that helps you out of your funk when you're at your lowest point.

Your "why" needs to be stronger than all of your excuses.

When you find your "why," it will be only a matter of time before you reach your goals—it's that important! By understanding your "why," you can maximise your potential

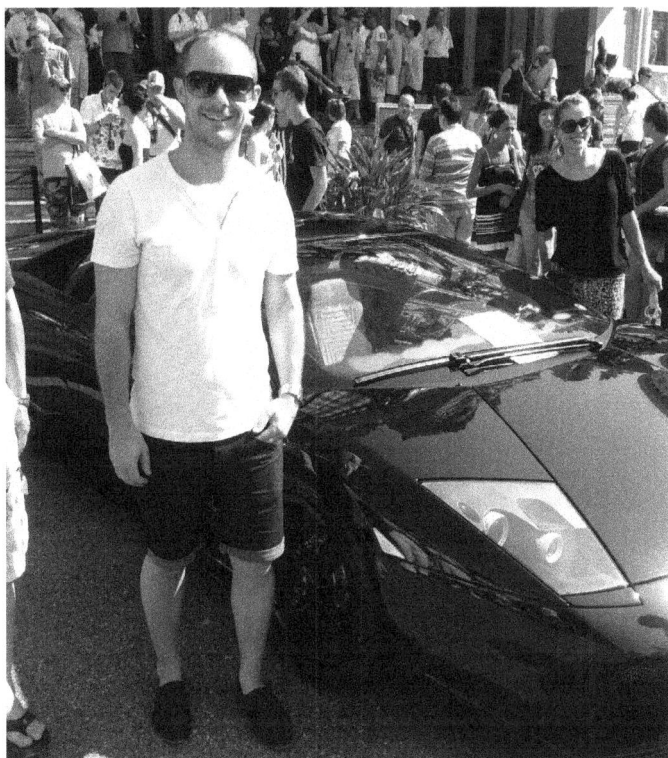

and well-being. Knowing and acting on your "why" is a powerful guiding force that requires an extremely strong emotional commitment. Having said that, however, it's unlikely that you'll attain any of your goals without being happy first.

I always approach health and weight loss with happiness at the forefront of my mind because, as we discovered in the previous chapter, fitness isn't just for abs. Too many people think having the body of their dreams or losing a certain amount of weight will give them happiness, but if you talk to the best-looking supermodels on the planet, they'll still bad-mouth their own bodies. It's this never-ending journey of trying to find a perfect body because that'll mean you've then found happiness, but that's simply not true. Happiness is a choice. Be happy with yourself, and the rest will follow.

If your "happiness end goal" is having the perfect body or being a certain weight, you will never achieve real happiness, because as soon as you get there, you'll find something else you don't like about yourself. You'll then alter your vision of the perfect body and work toward that. It never ends, and you're never actually happy.

Acknowledging what makes you happy *right at this moment* will set you up for success in reaching your fitness goal, or any goals for that matter. When we are happy—when our mind-set and mood are positive—we are smarter, more motivated, and thus more successful. Happiness is the center, and success revolves around it. When our brains fall stuck in a pattern that focuses on stress and negativity, we set ourselves up to fail. Undoing negative patterns and establishing positive ones is key.

I will give you an example. Like most men, I want to look good on the beach, so I perform a lot of exercises to make my biceps bigger and so on. This is definitely an important part of my life, but I would sacrifice my biceps and the desire to look physically pleasing in a heartbeat if it meant spending more time with my family. For me, happiness is spending time with my family because they're important to me. Spending time with them also alleviates my stresses. If I'm less stressed, I'm a better father, husband, and person. This then motivates me to exercise, which then leads to weight loss as a secondary benefit. If I'm not spending time with my family, I'll stress out and spend too much time at work, which cuts even more time away from my loved ones; and then exercise and weight loss become inconsequential, and I don't care about them. This, of course, then leads to unhealthy eating habits and weight gain.

It's a vicious cycle that most people perpetuate because their sole focus is to get a "perfect body" that they think will make them happy, which is the wrong way of looking at it. Find that happiness in yourself right now. For me, as I said, it's spending quality time with my family. For others, it could be going on a vacation once a month, or being outside, or reading. Whatever it might be, you need to find happiness within yourself. Finding whatever makes you happy and focusing on it will certainly set you up for success in your health journey.

The never-ending pursuits of "I need to earn more," or "I need to have a big house," or "I need to look great" are society-imposed ideas. These are long-established milestones that society has equated with success and therefore happiness—things we've been taught to aim for. I've been a product of that thought process myself. I thought I needed to drive a fancy car and live in a big house in order to be happy. It's only recently that I've thought much more about this idea of happiness and that you must find it within yourself first (although I still want that Lambo!).

SUSTAINABILITY AND QUALITY OF LIFE

People don't stick with lifestyle changes over time without two essential elements: sustainability and a quality of life.

Traditional fasts and the 5:2 diet dictate fasting for a full day, which is incredibly difficult for the average person. Unless you practise regular fasts as a part of your culture or religion, fasting for a full day is too disruptive to our lives and thus a detriment to our quality of life. If I tell you to fast all day on Fridays and Mondays, and then your best mate calls you up and says, "Hey, you want to go out for drinks Friday night?" you won't want to say, "Oh, sorry. I'm fasting today, I can't come out for drinks." It disrupts your lifestyle too much to stick to it long-term.

You might be able to get away with it for a little while and say, "Sorry, mate. I'm fasting," but at some point, you'll crack. Skipping breakfast as stage one in the Start Late, Stay Light lifestyle doesn't disrupt your quality of life, and it's sustainable because it's not as restrictive as other diets. Instead, it focuses on *when* to eat rather than *what* to eat, which is far easier and less disruptive. My biggest gripe with most fad diets is they prohibit eating our favourite foods—and no body wants that.

Now don't get me wrong. If you look good in a bikini and have "that perfect body," I'm not trying to insinuate that your quality of life is bad. In order to be ripped and have the movie-star body, however, you're probably eating a restricted diet, meaning you might not go out with friends or have much of a social life. And if that's your thing, great! I think it all comes back to what your goals are, your "why," and what makes you happy. If your goals are to be on stage in a bikini competition, you're going to make certain sacrifices to get into that kind of shape, which I don't think most of us are prepared to do.

In my experience, most people want to feel healthy and be in a normal weight range. They want to be able to move, run, and play with their kids and grandkids. They don't want to lose their breath climbing stairs. They want to be able to get back up if they fall down. Quality of life comes from being able to enjoy family holidays and hanging out with your best mates on Friday nights. If you're a healthy person—and this doesn't mean you have the biggest biceps or that bikini body—and you can run and hike with your kids even as an older person, then I think your quality of life is much better than the person who won Mr. Olympia this year.

Later-day eating is not a diet; it's a lifestyle. It's not a diet, because it doesn't change or restrict the foods you want to eat. It's the easiest way to change people's eating habits without drastically interrupting their lives. And again, people can choose any diet plan or food pathway they want as a layer within the Start Late, Stay Light lifestyle. You can be gluten-free, paleo, or sugar-free—it doesn't matter. This lifestyle can work for you.

The beauty of later-day eating is you can have it 100 percent customised. One of the many questions I ask my clients up front is, "What food could you never live without?" and I always make sure to fit that favourite food within the food plan I create for them. It's often a fun conversation.

"You mean I can enjoy ice cream every single night, and I'm going to lose weight?"

"Yep."

"I don't believe you."

"Just follow the program, and I guarantee you'll see results."

Three to four weeks later, they're posting pictures on the Start Late, Stay Light Facebook page saying, "Look what I'm eating tonight (picture of ice cream), and I've lost three kilos!"

I asked my sister, Sarah, the same question at the start of her journey. Her answer: "On Friday night, I love eating a burger and some ice cream." She's certainly not alone in enjoying high-calorie meals like burgers and ice cream. In creating her meal plan, I searched for lower-calorie ice creams that were still tasty. It took some work to find alternatives, but I did it, and now every Friday night, she knows a burger and ice cream is on the menu, and she doesn't feel guilty about it whatsoever.

The most common answers people give me are "I love chocolate," or, "I love bread," or, "I love pasta." We can make all of those work so you never feel like you're going without.

THE FOLLOWING CHAPTERS

I'm going to give you everything you need to know about the Start Late, Stay Light lifestyle; the ideas underlying the program are broken up and presented in five stages. In the following chapters, I'll tell you what you need to know (backed up by science of course!) and how to implement each stage. The further along you progress, the more changes you will see.

Stage one is breaking through the breakfast myth.

Stage two is understanding energy in, energy out.

Stage three is dedicated to the importance of protein, the king of macronutrients.

Stage four is dedicated to the other two macronutrients, carbohydrates and fats.

Stage five is about incorporating movement and tying it all together.

At the end of all the chapters, you'll find my entire sixteen-week program (one for males and one for females) for you to follow on your own. As you go through it, reference back to the chapter that coincides with each stage to help you. Give it a go on your own, but if you need extra help,

I'm here for you. In fact, if you've read this far, despite my publisher advising against this, I want you to email me (info@startlatestaylight.com) so I can personally email you back and give you a little gift to say thank you.

When you get to stage five, you should be coming to the end of the sixteen-week program in the back pages of the book. Once you get there, be sure to congratulate yourself for becoming an official later-day eater! Don't forget to send me your transformation pictures with a big beaming smile to show me how happy you are with the results and tell me how you feel!

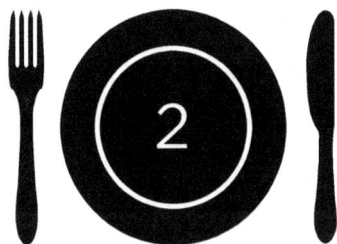

STAGE ONE: BREAKING THROUGH THE KELLOGG'S MYTH

Fasting has been promoted and practised worldwide from antiquity, by physicians, by the founders and followers of many religions, by culturally designated individuals, and by individuals or groups as an expression of protest against what they believe are violations of social, ethical, or political principles. In recent years, fasting has made its mark in the health and fitness world, and not only as a way to lose weight and build muscle. New research is emerging every day that supports fasting as a way to help manage or prevent certain diseases and conditions.

FASTING FOR WEIGHT LOSS

In order to understand how you can lose weight while fasting, you need to understand some basic facts about the metabolism. Glucose and fat are the body's main sources of energy. If glucose is not available, then the body will adjust by using fat.[1] It takes most people twelve to fourteen hours for their body to burn the majority of the sugar stored in their body as glycogen. Once the glycogen stores in your liver and muscles are practically depleted, your body searches for an alternate energy source, so it turns to its fat stores. It's at this point that you start to lose weight and glean a bunch of other health benefits (more on that later). Most people, however, never reach this point, as they eat as soon as they wake up and continue to eat meals throughout the day on the assumption that it raises their metabolism. This thus teaches their body to burn sugar as its primary fuel and effectively shuts off its ability to use fat as a fuel.

The reality is that fasting is an intrinsic part of human life. Congratulations! You're already practising intermittent fasting—its most basic form is called sleeping.

All of us fast when we sleep, which is roughly eight hours, give or take. And most of us eat our last meal a few hours

1   Jason Fung, "Fasting Physiology: Part II," Intensive Dietary Management, April 17, 2015, https://intensivedietarymanagement.com/fasting-physiology-part-ii/

before climbing into bed, increasing the fasting window a bit longer. By skipping breakfast and making lunch your first meal of the day, you're increasing your daily fasting time to sixteen hours or possibly even longer—well over the minimum amount required to shift into fat-burning mode. If you go longer than sixteen hours, you simply extend this process.

I am fully aware that we are different than mice; however, there was a study done with mice where two sets of mice were given the exact same amount of calories per day, but one set of mice received food throughout the day—eating breakfast, lunch, and dinner—and the other set of mice were restricted to a certain window of eating, fasting for about sixteen hours before receiving their first meal. The mice that fasted for sixteen hours a day weighed less, stayed healthy, and performed better when they exercised.

Keep in mind that while most people will successfully switch over to burning fat after several weeks of intermittent fasting, you may need several months to teach your body to turn on the fat-burning enzymes that allow your body to effectively use fat as its primary fuel.

Skipping breakfast is good for weight loss because it eliminates one meal right off the bat. Most breakfasts are around 400 to 700 calories. Those who need to lose weight are typically told to reduce their calories by 500 into a deficit; and the easiest way to do that, in my opinion, is to eliminate a meal—a meal that is nowhere near as important as we have been led to believe.

Take a look at some popular meals people eat for breakfast. Whether they are considered "good" or "bad," each one of them contains between 400 and 700 calories, which doesn't leave you with many left over for the remainder of the day.

Pancakes with Yoghurt, Fresh Fruit, and Maple Syrup

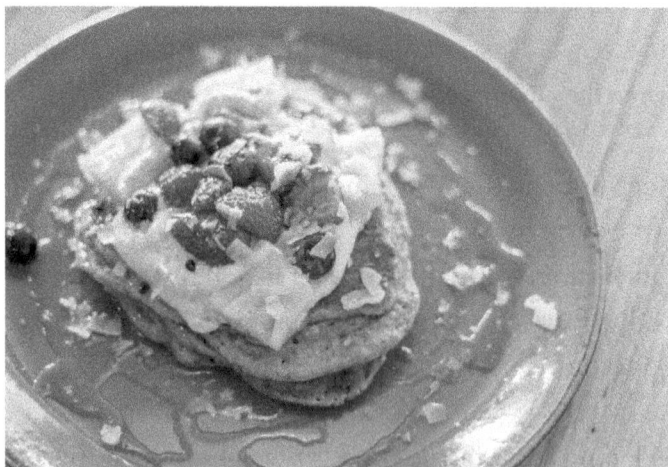

2 Pancakes (350)

50 g Blueberries (30)

50 g Strawberries (15)

100 g Fat-Free Yoghurt (52)

Drizzle of Maple Syrup (80)

Total Calories: 527 calories

Poached Eggs with Avocado and Feta

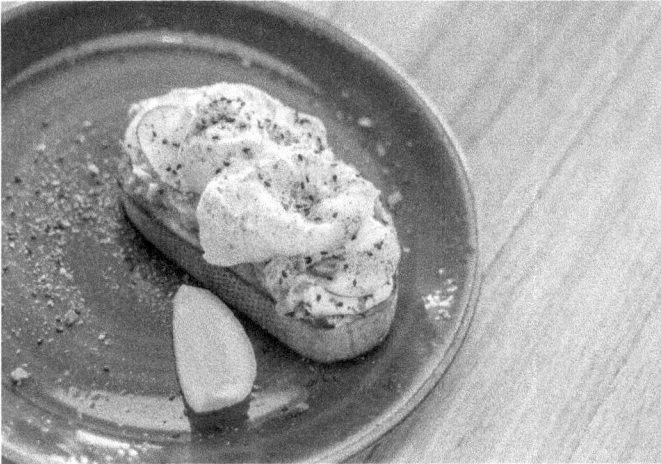

1 Slice of Rye Toast (120)

Butter on Toast (50)

2 Poached Eggs (136)

50 g Avocado (80)

Sprinkle of Feta (120)

Total Calories: 506 calories

Muesli with Yoghurt and Fresh Fruit

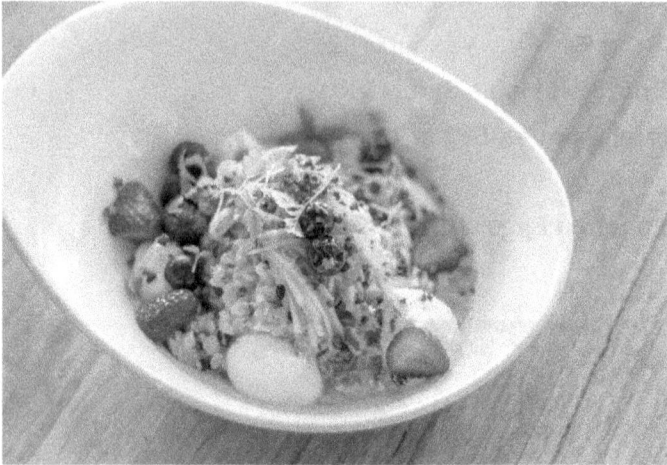

100 g Toasted Muesli (430)

250 ml Low Fat Milk (125)

100 g Fat-Free Yoghurt (52)

50 g Blueberries (30)

50 g Strawberries (15)

Total: 652 calories

Scrambled Eggs and Bacon with Grilled Tomato

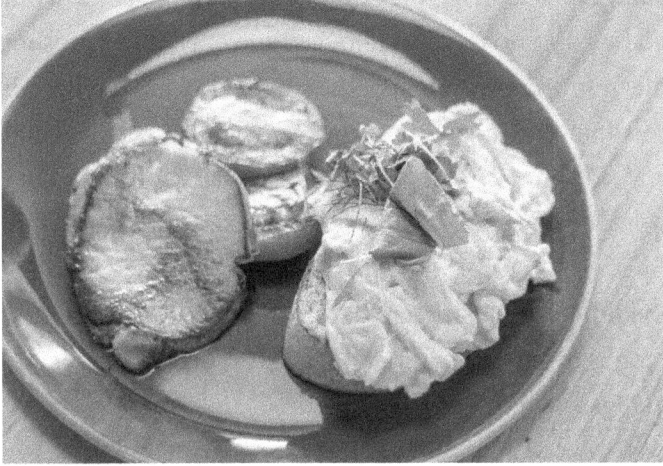

3 large eggs scrambled (210)
3 strips of bacon (138)
1 Slice of Rye Toast (120)
Butter on Toast (50)
Grilled Tomato (25)
Total: 543 calories

What I've found with my clients is that most of them want big and satisfying meals, so instead of reducing calories and splitting them among four or five small meals throughout the day, by getting rid of one big meal in the morning, they can have two standard-size (or even sometimes bigger) meals at the end of the day.

HORMONE BALANCE

WARNING: I reference a lot of science in the next few paragraphs to help you understand what happens in our bodies. I'm no endocrinologist, however, and I present this information to you based on my own research, so if you don't care about the science behind all this, go ahead and skip ahead. Rest assured that it's all good stuff, but I won't be offended if it doesn't interest you.

Evidence suggests that fasting also helps balance hormones that assist in the weight-loss process, specifically in regards to cortisol, testosterone, and estrogen.

Cortisol has many functions, but it's mostly known as the stress hormone. Its main purpose is to manage stress in the body, but it also helps the body use glucose and fat for energy. Levels of cortisol rise during tension-filled times, which causes higher insulin levels. When our blood sugar drops again, we typically crave sugary, fatty foods. Cortisol imbalances can turn your overeating into a habit.

When it comes to weight loss, cortisol is an absolute enemy because it inhibits a lot of the things that help us lose weight. That's why, in the first chapter, I stress the importance of finding happiness first. If you go into a calorie-restriction of any kind, even in my program, it's never an enjoyable thing. While I believe that my version of losing weight is certainly the easiest way to do it, when you're in a calorie-restricted state, your cortisol levels will inherently go up due to an increased level of stress. If you have other stresses in your life, whether that's work-related or you're in a bad relationship, cortisol continues to rise, and it'll make losing weight that much more difficult, so you want your overall state of mind to be positive.

Testosterone is one of many hormones that is responsible for muscle growth and muscle repair. Intermittent fasting increases testosterone, and it stimulates all the right hormones that support healthy testosterone production while suppressing the hormones that interfere with it. Every time you eat, your testosterone levels go down. Both men and women have levels of testosterone, but men naturally have more of it. Testosterone is the main reason why men are naturally bigger and have an easier time putting on muscle than women. That's why when you see females using steroids, the hormone testosterone goes through the roof, and they get a lot of male-like characteristics. Fasting increases your levels of testosterone (it doesn't come close to reaching the levels seen in steroids, so don't worry about growing a beard, girls) as well as human growth hormone (HGH). Research presented at the 2011 annual scientific sessions of the American College of Cardiology in New Orleans showed that fasting triggered a 1,300 percent rise of HGH in women, and an astounding 2,000 percent rise in men. HGH, commonly referred to as the "fitness hormone," plays an important role in maintaining health, fitness, and longevity, including promoting muscle growth and boosting fat loss by revving up your metabolism.

Fasting also affects estrogen levels. Just like testosterone, both men and women have levels of estrogen, but women tend to carry more of it. We have estrogen receptors throughout our bodies, including in our brains, GI tract, and bones. When we change our estrogen balance, we change metabolic function all over: cognition, moods, digestion, recovery, protein turnover, bone formation, and so on. When it comes to appetite and energy balance, estrogen works in a few ways. First, in the brain stem, estrogens modify the peptides that signal you to feel full (cholecystokinin) or hungry (ghrelin). In the hypothalamus, estrogens also stimulate neurons that halt production of appetite-regulating peptides. Estrogens are thus key metabolic regulators.[2]

In addition, your body collects a number of harmful agents as you go about your day. Due to the consistent demand of digestion, your body doesn't get the appropriate time it needs to engage in detoxification, and when

2 Hormone Health Network, "What Is Estrogen?", accessed February 12, 2017, http://www.hormone.org/diseases-and-conditions/womens-health/what-is-estrogen

you fast for a period of sixteen or more hours, your body has the time to do some positive "housekeeping." In a study published in the *American Journal of Physiology*, fasting increased the efficiency of the removal of toxins and estrogenic compounds.

CALORIES IN, CALORIES OUT

At the end of the day, weight loss happens when we consume fewer calories than we exude—*period*. There are also other factors that will alter how much weight you lose, depending on your level of deficit. That's why we don't always see a linear result when I give you and Bob a 500-calorie deficit; you may lose more weight than he does. Everyone's body loses weight differently, and there are other factors that determine the speed in which you lose weight. In general, though, if you want to lose weight, you have to be in a deficit consistently over a long period of time. The more you're in a deficit, the more weight you will lose.

If you can do that for long enough—*which is the key point and the main challenge for most people*—you are guaranteed to see results. Unfortunately, even the people who are capable of sustaining a calorie deficit often give up after only a few weeks. They don't allow enough time to pass and grow discouraged with the up-and-down fluctuations that commonly occur along their fitness journey. Weight loss isn't something that happens over ten weeks, as much as TV shows like *The Biggest Loser* might make it seem. If you can be in a deficit for long enough—six months, twelve months, eighteen months—you will see results, 100 percent certainly.

There's not a person on this planet who won't lose weight if they stay in a deficit long enough. I'm willing to lay my professional integrity on that.

The prime example of this are shows like *Survivor*, where guys and girls are on an island and they only eat rice—of course they're going to drop weight (side note: I have watched every single episode of this show, and one of my life's dreams is to be a participant, so if you are reading this, Jeff Probst, hook me up!). They all waste away because they're on the island for thirty days basically eating nothing. Another example of this, on the absolute extreme side, is prisoners of war. The Jews sent to concentration camps during World War II wasted away because they barely received any food. Their bodies were subjected to an extremely low-calorie diet and then forced to do vast amounts of heavy labour for a long period of time.

These days, a lot of diet companies need to market products that are sexy to the consumer, which usually means using lingo like, "Lose ten kilos in ten days." Newsflash, people: If losing weight were easy, everyone would do it and succeed—but it's not easy. Most products you see advertised all try to do the same thing: restrict the way you consume calories. I'm not saying my program is going to be easy, because weight loss takes discipline, dedication, and hard work, but it's certainly a simplified way to rid some calories out of your diet.

FASTING FOR OTHER HEALTH BENEFITS

One of the primary mechanisms that makes intermittent fasting so beneficial for health is related to its impact on your insulin sensitivity. While sugar is a source of energy for your body, it also promotes insulin resistance when consumed in the amounts found in our modern processed food diets. Insulin resistance, in turn, is a primary driver of chronic disease—from heart disease to cancer. Mounting research confirms that when your body becomes accustomed to burning fat instead of sugar as its primary fuel, you dramatically reduce your risk of chronic disease. Becoming fat adapted may even be a key strategy for both cancer prevention and treatment, as cancer cells cannot utilise fat for fuel—they need *sugar* to thrive.

Research has found that after a few hours of fasting (which technically starts after that twelve-hour mark), our bodies starts to burn fat and break down cholesterol into beneficial bile acids, once our bodies exhaust their stores of readily available energy. These beneficial bile acids basically flip that fuel-switch selector, so instead of using glycogen in the body, it starts using fat. The liver, meanwhile, shuts down the glucose production for several hours, which then lowers your blood glucose levels. The extra glucose is used to repair damaged cells and also make new DNA, which can help prevent chronic inflammation. Liver enzymes that are also activated help in the creation of brown fat, and this is the good kind, which converts into extra calories via heat.

Fasting has also been shown to reduce cholesterol.

DON'T EAT IN THE MORNING

Now that you're familiar with all the amazing reasons why fasting can help you, the first step in my program is simple: Stop eating breakfast—which means stop eating in the morning. That's as simple as it gets. Don't think about anything else. Don't worry about the calories you're eating throughout the rest of the day or what you're eating, *for now*. Just do what you usually do, but don't start eating until around 1:00 p.m., depending on when you last ate the night before; make sure you fast for sixteen hours.

Step two: Don't freak out.

Most people tend to freak out about stage one because they're worried they'll get incredibly hungry in the morning. If you've fallen for the "breakfast is the most important meal of the day" trap and have subsequently always eaten breakfast, then it might be a bit of a challenge for you in the beginning. Don't fret, though! Turns out, it's mostly a mental challenge, and most people end up skipping it cold turkey and do just fine.

Caffeine is allowed in the morning, as long as it's straight black coffee. Coffee without any additives (sugar, cream, milk, etc.) has zero calories, so you can drink it—I usually don't recommend more than two to three cups though.

Caffeine is a fantastic appetite suppressant, so if you like the taste of coffee, I highly encourage you to drink it in the morning to help you get through to your first meal. I'm personally not a coffee drinker; I never have been. I don't like the smell or taste of it (I also have a bet going with my mum that I won't before the age of fifty). I'm up at 4:30 a.m. and in the office by 5:30 a.m. every day, and most of my team members have coffee in hand, stinking up the whole place—it makes me feel ill. I understand, however, that most people are coffee fans, so go ahead and enjoy your cup as long as it doesn't have any extra calories in it.

You can't add sugar or milk, which bums most people out because they love their lattes or cappuccinos.

I think most people these days like coffee because it has become a habit. I'd encourage those latte and cappuccino drinkers to find great quality and learn to appreciate the flavour of actual coffee. Find talented baristas who know their craft and get some insight on quality beans, where they come from, and how coffee should be enjoyed. I say if you're going to do something, do it correctly. (Please don't drink Starbucks, either—it's not real coffee! I know this could have been a big chance to garner a sponsor and make millions by being tied to Starbucks, but I think it's plain garbage, and I don't want you drinking it!) A better quality, stronger coffee has more benefits with regards to appetite suppression due to the amount of caffeine. Most people on my program usually drink two cups of coffee before their first meal, and those latte coffee drinkers reported that it only took a week or two to grow accustomed to drinking coffee black.

If you're not a coffee person and you prefer tea in the morning, that's completely fine as well, but the same rules apply: no sugar or milk. Only drink teas with zero calories. There are some herbal teas with certain additives that have calories, so watch out for those. Most teas have zero calories, though, and they are absolutely okay to drink during your morning fast.

I typically only drink water in the mornings, but every once in a while I'll need a boost of some sort. If it's been a long night with the baby, for example, I'll drink a Monster Zero, an energy drink with zero calories (hint, hint, Monster, I think you should sponsor me!). Since I don't touch caffeine on a regular basis, after drinking one of those, I bounce off the walls, and I literally cannot stop talking. And since those things have the equivalent amount of caffeine as three coffees in it, that caffeinated energy lasts for a good ten hours. It has zero calories, though, so I'm not breaking my fast!

Hydration is essential during your morning fast, especially for caffeine drinkers. Caffeine is a diuretic, causing dehydration, so be sure you drink plenty of water throughout your mornings. I don't think people drink enough water as it is, so getting in that hydration is essential—and it'll help you with those hunger pangs. The first couple of days, when new clients hit 10:00 a.m., they get pretty hungry because their bodies are conditioned to have eaten something at that point. Having fluid in your stomach can certainly stave off that hungry kind of pain you feel in your stomach. If you follow me on Snapchat (and you should because I'm hugely entertaining!—my username is StartLate) my first snap every morning is of me drinking a big bottle of water. I'm serious. I post the exact same snap every day because I am a man who believes you should practise what you preach.

If you drink anything with calories in it, you've broken your fast, and your body won't reach that critical moment of using fat storage for energy use, so don't drink anything with calories in it until after your sixteen-hour marker. And since we're on the topic, you should never drink anything that has calories in it—it's such a waste! Before sipping on anything, look up the calories. Juices, soda, and alcohol, to name a few, are *full* of calories that you can use on delicious food (like ice cream!). That juice you thought was a good option and drank this morning has more calories in it than a glass of coke!

HABITS CAN BE BROKEN

Hunger in the morning is a habit, and like all habits, it can be broken. When you play tennis week in and week out, you become a better tennis player. Eating breakfast is ingrained in us from a young age, so it's hard to break a habit that you've held for the majority of your life. You probably have a positive association with breakfast, too, making it an even harder habit to break. Perhaps you shared big breakfasts with your family every Sunday as a kid growing up. Or maybe your mum made you pancakes when you were feeling sad. I think hunger, most of the time, is more psychological than it is physical. Even though you think you're hungry in the morning, that hunger mostly comes from the habit you've developed over the years. And like breaking other habits, there are different ways to do so. If you're a smoker, for example, there are various methods to stop smoking. The same thing can be said for quitting breakfast, too. You can either do it cold turkey or take it slowly. Perhaps instead of eating breakfast at 8:00 a.m. as you normally would, you can start eating breakfast at 10:00 a.m. for a week or two. Then extend it again to noon or 1:00 p.m. the following week. Find whatever works for you. Most people find it pretty easy to go cold turkey, though.

As if skipping breakfast and breaking a habit isn't hard enough, you'll also encounter outside opposition to your new endeavor. More likely than not, you'll have plenty of people telling you that you are doing your body harm and that you should eat something—don't listen to them! They more than likely don't have any qualification to tell you that it's a bad or a good thing. Heck, I have people in my own profession telling me I am irresponsible for writing this book. People will always tell you their opinion, which will make this even harder; be strong, remember your "why," and keep going!

If you don't work a regular nine-to-five schedule, it doesn't matter. Simply adjust so that you're fasting for sixteen hours out of your day. I had a client who worked the night shift and slept during the day, so his timeline was a little different. The time of day means nothing; it's the timing of when you eat.

Once you've made it to that sixteen-hour mark, eat as you normally would. During this stage, I want you to focus on skipping breakfast; don't focus too much on anything else. It's important to break the habit of eating breakfast, since that is the foundation of my Start Late, Stay Light lifestyle. Eating normally may even involve drinking alcohol or eating fast food, and that's okay. As I've already mentioned, by not eating breakfast, you're automatically eliminating 500 or more calories out of your diet. Five hundred calories every day over the course of a week is 3,500 calories, which equates to almost half a kilo.

More likely than not, you're going to see weight loss even if you change nothing else in the short-term. Don't get too excited though: that's only going to last until you stabilise what your daily intake should be. During the first few weeks in stage one, all you need to do is skip breakfast. We'll start fine-tuning the program as we move along and reach other stages.

There are people who claim that if you skip breakfast, you'll eat more during the rest of the day to compensate. And although there are a few people who might do this, in general, this is inaccurate. *The New Scientist*, a highly regarded journal, conducted a study to see if this would happen, and they found that people did not overcompensate eating if they skipped breakfast. The study fed a 700-calorie breakfast to the group who were having breakfast and then tracked how many calories they ate for the rest of the day. They then looked at the group that skipped breakfast and also tracked the calories they consumed from their first meal until their last. They didn't control what either group ate after breakfast. The people who didn't have breakfast did eat a slightly bigger lunch and a slightly bigger dinner, but those extra calories never made up the 700 calories the first group ate for breakfast. The group that fasted might have enjoyed an extra 100 calories over lunchtime and then an extra 150 calories at dinner; however, the people who ate breakfast ate in total more calories throughout the entire day.

THE KELLOGG'S MYTH

Breakfast wasn't always about a healthy start. Historically if you had a hard day ahead of you doing manual labour on the farm, it made sense to fuel your body with a good breakfast. The idea of health wasn't a consideration; it focused on fueling for the day ahead on a labour-intensive farm.

Then came the Industrial Revolution, and our days became less physical and the need for refueling less obvious. It was around the turn of the last century when Dr. John Harvey Kellogg popped up with his cereal, which revolutionised the idea of breakfast as being healthy. Dr. Kellogg, a devout Seventh-day Adventist, invented his cornflakes because he thought that eating pure, wholesome food would stop people from masturbating.

I'm not kidding.

This guy was something else. Apparently, he never had sex with his wife. They adopted all their kids since he thought sex was a thing of the devil. He wanted to come up with something that would keep people from masturbating, so he came up with a lie to market to the public promoting fibre as a way to decrease masturbation. Here's an excerpt I read from the *News Scientist Journal*.

> *As a doctor, he also believed that the common health concerns of the day, like digestion and regularity, could be improved by consuming his fibrous cornflakes. Kellogg managed to take these free-floating health anxieties and embody them in a product. Both the product and*

the concept were well received. People hadn't had health food marketed to them before. Women, who traditionally cooked a large breakfast for their family, thought it was a godsend. Convinced this new cereal was "healthier" for their families took the guilt away from buying breakfast in a box. It was such a successful marketing vehicle that others piggybacked onto it. Other staples of our breakfast routine, including orange juice and coffee, then followed. The popularity of bacon for breakfast was allegedly the brainchild of Edward Bernays, the self-styled grandfather of public relations. In the 1920s, he was commissioned by the U.S. pork industry to boost bacon sales. Bernays surveyed medical doctors and asked them one question: Is a hearty breakfast preferable? It had nothing to do with health. He just asked if it was preferable. The resounding answer of course was yes. Presumably as a relic of the ideas of breakfast and refueling from a bygone agricultural days, Bernays used this fact in marketing campaigns and the popularity of bacon and eggs went through the roof. I'm not trying to trash the benefits of breakfast all together, but it's safe to say the idea that it is healthy on its own was laid on a plate for us by a marketing company and by large we've gobbled it up ever since.

The Kellogg's company today, like most companies, relies on our buying its products. If we all stopped eating breakfast, they'd go out of business. They're there for profits, not for our health.

When you look at the research that's gone into our eating habits and our health benefits, a lot of it is funded by the food companies. The government then publishes its recommended daily intakes for what we should be doing, based on many of these findings.

Unfortunately, this happens all the time. Some company will fund research that says eating their product is better for you, but in reality, they're only saying that so they stay in business. I'm a big skeptic when I see something advertised on TV. Is [insert product here] really good for me? Even these days, on social-media platforms like Instagram and Snapchat, there are so many people who have a huge following—one to one hundred million followers—and companies will approach them and ask them to endorse one of their products, paying top dollar if they say yes. I am dead against this. There are many fitness influencers these days who are paid $1,000 or more per post by companies to promote their products—products they probably don't even use or believe in, but they don't care. Why should they? They're being paid. In my opinion, it's dirty marketing. In most cases, they're not doing it because they want to help us; they're doing it because they are being paid. I know I joked earlier about wanting companies to sponsor me, but I have never—and I will never—pushed a product in exchange for money. If I like something, I'll tell you I like it because I like it, not because I have been paid to tell you so. Products I do showcase on my social-media platforms are products I find valuable and use every day.

That's why I have a big gripe with the breakfast industry as well. There is little evidence suggesting eating breakfast is good for your health. It was purely a marketing ploy, and we've stuck with it ever since. No one's ever questioned it because it is so ingrained into us. So many doctors sit on it, too, and when doctors are telling to you to do something, you're obviously going to do it since doctors are usually highly regarded and you trust them.

The truth of the matter is that we are better off not eating breakfast because most breakfasts are full of sugar anyway. However, I'm advocating never eating a sugary breakfast cereal again. If you can't live without your favourite breakfast cereals, eat them after your sixteen-hour fast. If you love cornflakes, have them for lunch. I love Froot Loops, for example. For me, this cereal reminds me of when I was a little kid. For my birthday, my mum used to let me choose whatever cereal I wanted, and I always went for Froot Loops—and it brings up good memories. Nowadays, I use cereal for when I'm in a bulking phase. I need quite a lot of carbohydrates per day on training days, and to get that amount of carbohydrates from "clean sources" like potatoes, vegetables, and fruit is near impossible. You'd have to eat kilos and kilos of them to get enough in, whereas I can get a huge amount of carbohydrates from a bowl of cereal because it's full of sugar. One bowl of Fruit Loops nets me 80 to 100 grams of carbohydrates fairly easily, whereas I would have to eat more than half a kilo of potatoes to reach the same level. Just know that the morning is certainly not the place to enjoy sugary breakfast foods.

After only a few days of skipping breakfast, people have reported an increase in energy, an increase in focus, and no midmorning or afternoon crashes. I tend to book all my clients in the morning, workout at lunchtime, and then go home for a bite to eat. This has been my routine for years. Since skipping breakfast, I've found I feel much more energised to do my afternoon workout than I used to.

There are studies that seem to suggest subjects also cognitively perform better. They'll give you a task of remembering twenty items in the morning, and if you're the non-breakfast eater and I'm the breakfast eater, and we get retested at lunchtime, it turns out my level of remembering those things would be worse than yours. These cognitive studies show that people who skip breakfast are more alert, more switched on, and perform better during exercise.

It makes sense if you think about it. Looking back to our caveman DNA and genetics again, a caveman wouldn't kill a deer and then bring it back to the cave every night for his wife to cook him a nice big feast. They only ever ate when they caught their food, which definitely wasn't an everyday occurrence. More often than not, their bodies were in fasted states for quite some time until they successfully did find, hunt, and kill an animal. It doesn't make sense for our bodies to start shutting down and being less effective or less efficient at hunting and gathering, because if that were the case, we'd probably all have died out. The body doesn't want to die, so instead, it thinks, "I'd better be more heightened and more alert." In a state of stress, especially when it ignites the fight-or-flight response, your body kicks into high gear with sharper hearing, better vision, and more focus and energy in order to survive. Scientists credit the higher energy level after fasting with the fact that it's been built into us.

I've also found that I sleep better after concentrating my meals toward the end of the day, as we are suited to sleep with a full belly. It suits our genetics because in caveman days we would've gone a day or days without food, and when we would have finally killed something, put it on the fire, and ate a huge feast, our digestive systems would be at work and we would sleep well, no longer needing to be alert to hunt. I sleep much better after big meals compared to when I eat smaller portions throughout the day.

When I used to eat breakfast, I would experience a midmorning crash where I felt I needed some sort of pick-me-up. Perhaps you fall into this category as well. You're at work, and come midmorning, you can't keep your eyes open. After skipping breakfast, I don't experience crashes anymore, and a lot of my clients report the same thing, explaining that they have a much more stable energy level throughout the day. This has to do with your glucose levels, which we covered previously. If you have a big meal in the morning, your glucose levels go through the roof, and insulin is released. Once your body uses that as energy, your body feels tired and your brain sends you signals that you need a pick-me-up again.

Stage one of simply skipping breakfast is what I want you to concentrate on for the first four weeks. You might hit some bumps in the road in the beginning, but after only a few days, your body will accept your changes, and you will immediately see some exciting changes.

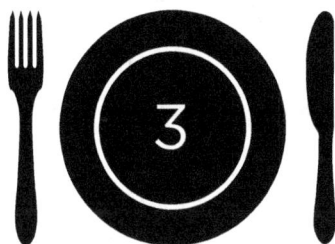

STAGE TWO: ENERGY IN, ENERGY OUT

In order to lose weight, we have to burn more calories than we consume. Energy in, energy out—it's as simple as that. Contrary to some common lore, certain foods don't burn calories; it's the lean muscle tissue, brain, and organs in your body that are responsible for using energy. Now, before you flood my email inbox correcting me, yes, there is a thermic effect of food; however, it is extremely small compared to what our bodies, systems, and lean muscle tissue burns on a daily basis. That's why I promote protein as an essential part of this whole equation (more on that later). The more lean muscle mass you have—that is, muscles—the more energy your body needs to be alive.

I'll give you an example. Two men both weigh 100 kilos, but one guy has 10% body fat and the second guy has 40% fat. The first guy is a bodybuilder, and at 10% body fat, he has 90 kilos of lean muscle tissue. The second guy is overweight, unhealthy, and at 40% body fat, he has only 60 kilos of lean muscle tissue. Even though they're both 100 kilos, the first guy is going to use a lot more energy per day to fuel his body than the second guy. That's where the "energy in, energy out" balance is different because the first guy needs to eat a lot more food to fuel his body than the second guy.

The basic law of thermodynamics is energy in equals energy out. Unfortunately, this basic law is not sexy sounding. If I'm on the TV saying, "I have the secret to help you lose weight," and then I follow that up with, "Just stop eating as much," it's not sexy, it's not fancy, and it's not exciting. But that is the secret: Energy in equals energy out. If you follow this law for long enough and you're consistent, it will work—it's that simple.

Regardless of muscle mass, we all use energy, no matter what we're doing, even when we sleep. This is called your basal metabolic rate (BMR), and it's basically the number of calories you would burn if you stayed in bed all day. There are a lot of equations out there to work out your BMR, but there are only a couple that take into consideration your lean muscle mass. The one I've found to be the most accurate is the Katch-McArdle Method. I use it to determine all my clients' BMR, and it helps me decipher a lot of factors when I put together a meal and fitness plan. It provides a much more accurate estimate of how many calories you should be eating compared to other equations.

In order to perform this calculation, you must know your body fat percentage. You can guesstimate it by using a scale that will tell you your weight and body percent fat, or if you're looking for a more accurate reading, you could have a DEXA scan done. The Katch-McArdle equation uses the following formula to calculate BMR for both men and women:

BMR = 370 + (21.6 x Lean Mass in kilograms)

Just for fun, let's take the two men mentioned before and show you how different their BMRs would be. Bob weighs 100 kg with 40% body fat, and he has 60 kg of lean mass; so he would have a BMR of 370 + (21.6 x 60) = 1,666 calories per day.

John, on the other hand, who is also 100 kg, has 10% body fat and 90 kg of lean mass; so he would have a BMR of 370 + (21.6 x 90) = 2,314 calories. That's a massive difference!

Once you have determined your BMR, you must multiply it by the appropriate activity factor to determine your Total Daily Energy Expenditure or TDEE:

1.200 = sedentary (little or no exercise)
1.375 = light activity (light exercise/sports 1–3 days/week)
1.550 = moderate activity (moderate exercise/sports 3–5 days/week)
1.725 = super active (hard exercise/sports 6–7 days a week)
1.900 = extra active (intense exercise/sports and physical job)

That's all there is to it. Of course, if you want to avoid all of this arithmetic, simply visit www.StartLateStayLight.com or email me (info@startlatestaylight.com), and I will be happy to work out your estimated TDEE.

You should look at fitness as a science experiment, and it will take some time to perfect the formula for each individual. We figure out how many calories you need to eat, and then we test it out. After a few weeks, we assess progress and make any necessary changes. If you're gaining weight, then you're probably eating too much. If you're losing weight, and that's where you want to be heading, then the calculation was correct and you should keep going.

TRACK WHAT YOU EAT

Stage two is when we start tracking what we eat. It's the only way you're going to learn what's in your food and how to make long-term changes. And before you start whining and complaining that you hate tracking, know that you won't have to do it for the rest of your life. As a starting point, I have written out an entire meal plan for sixteen weeks, which you can find in the back of this book. There will come a point when you will be able to eye your meals and guesstimate the values without a tracker (like Neo, remember?), but you have to track for a period of time to get a feel for how many calories and macronutrients are in the foods you typically eat. Most of us eat the same foods over and over again throughout a course of five months or six months. Once you have enough practise, you won't have to always track. As you progress with your fitness, you'll likely have to return to tracking to adjust your input and output levels, but after a few weeks of doing so again, you'll be able to return to eyeballing and guestimating.

This is the stage where people start to fail at weight-loss programs because they don't want to put in the work. They're looking for that magic pill. Sorry, there isn't one; you have to suck it up and put in the effort. When you track your food, you learn about calorie input and output. It's the only way you're going to see long, sustainable results.

Good news though! Tracking today has never been easier! With a million different phone apps to choose from, there's no excuse not to track your food, especially since our phones are attached to our hips. When you eat something, simply pull out your phone, plug in your foods or scan the barcode, and bam! You're done. Easy! It's not like I'm asking you to carry a notepad with a pen around with you everywhere you go to jot down what you eat all day long. It's a much easier process to do these days, thanks to technology—so just do it.

MyFitnessPal is probably the most popular app out there. Remember Mike Vacanti whom I talked about earlier? Well, he created his own app, too, called Mike's Macros (previously called On the Regimen). It's also a great app that has a less extensive data base, but it is extremely accurate. There are a bunch of apps to choose from, but I recommend MyFitnessPal because it has such an extensive database of food and it's the app I use.

Be careful with MyFitnessPal, though, as the database has been created by users, and unfortunately, humans make mistakes, so some of the numbers for the food stored in the app are wrong. The cool thing, though, is you can add foods that aren't in the database, too. MyFitnessPal has a scanning feature so you can take your phone, scan the barcode of a food item, and then add it to the database.

The company itself also goes through and verifies certain products, making sure they are accurate. When you're using the app, you'll see a little green checkmark next to the verified food items, meaning the macronutrient numbers associated with those items are correct.

Since you'll be tracking your food, you'll need a kitchen scale so you can accurately weigh the foods you're eating (make sure to weigh your food in its raw or uncooked state). Again, this might not be a forever thing, but for those who have never tracked before, this is an essential part of the learning process. I always get some kickback from clients saying tracking with a weight scale is so pedantic and that it takes so much longer—but it's not, and it doesn't. I love using Snapchat stories (did I mention you should add me?—my username is StartLate) as a way to show how easy it is to measure food and how it takes an extra four seconds out of your day. It isn't as pedantic or time-consuming as people believe it is; don't be lazy. It's easy to throw a bowl on a scale and add in each food item to hit your numbers.

We've also been conditioned by restaurants to eat excessively large portions. We then bring those portions home and replicate them in our kitchens, so you're likely eating three times the amount you should be. Using a kitchen scale will open your eyes and teach you what proper portions look like, which is essential for your fitness journey. We've become so desensitised to exactly what a portion is these days because a lot of restaurants employ a "more is better" philosophy. If they give their customers a big meal, they'll come back, because a big meal is what people want. And on top of that, I think people also want to get their money's worth. If they're going to spend fifteen dollars on a burrito, the burrito better be big as hell.

WHAT SHOULD YOU EAT?

Your meal plan comes from your energy balance, meaning the amount of calories your body needs to survive, broken down into proteins, carbs, and fats. Once you've sorted your TDEE, let's figure out the macronutrient ratios that will make up your diet.

Here are the calorie values for each macronutrient again:

1 g Protein = 4 Calories
1 g Carbohydrate = 4 Calories
1 g Fat = 9 Calories

Ideally, you want to eat between 100 grams and a 180 grams of protein per day. Most people eat between 40 grams and 80 grams per day—yikes.

It works out to be about 0.6 to 0.7 grams per pound of body weight. If you're 200 pounds, multiply your weight by 0.6 or 0.7, and that equates to how much protein you should be eating at the lower end of the spectrum. If you are someone who is quite active, who only needs to lose a few kilos, and you don't have a lot of body fat, I'd probably have you somewhere down at the lower end of the range. If you have a higher body fat percentage and not a lot of muscle mass, then you'd probably start somewhere around the 1 to 1.2 grams per pound of body weight.

Once you've figured out how many calories of protein you need, 25–30 percent of your total calories should come from fats (more on the importance of fats later). The rest of the calories are given to carbohydrates. For example, a person who weighs 84 kilos and worked out a TDEE of 1,385 calories would need 130 grams of protein, which equals 520 calories. Twenty-five percent of this person's total calories are dedicated to fats, which would be 38 grams equaling 346 calories. This would leave 519 calories left to go to carbohydrates, which would equal 129 grams. You can always email me (info@startlatestaylight.com) if you'd like help.

Most people struggle with creating a meal plan for themselves in order to hit their numbers because they've never been taught how to eat properly. Tracking will fix this, but it will take time. Most people don't even come close to their protein numbers in the beginning, and they're eating too many fats and carbohydrates. With enough practise, however, you'll learn to balance your food intake.

This is often a huge challenge for people because they simply don't understand enough about food. How do I get my protein up? How do I keep my fats down? It takes a lot of trial and error. If you're a pure novice and you're lost with this whole tracking thing, jump onto my YouTube channel (Start Late, Stay Light) or my website (www.StartLateStayLight.com), where I answer a lot of questions and give away plenty of free content (I know, I know—shameless plugs everywhere; but I'm here to help!). Remember, you're a science experiment. The best way to figure out your meal plan is to give it a go. It's a matter of plugging things into MyFitnessPal and trying them. Start by inputting all the food you plan to eat for that day, and then look at the breakdown of proteins, carbs, and fats. If you're low on protein, return to the menu you created and see where you can make adjustments. Maybe you could add a protein shake. Maybe you'll add a little bit more chicken for lunch; rather than 100 grams, increase it to 150 grams. When you swap back to the breakdown of numbers, perhaps the protein levels have been fixed, but now your carbohydrates and fats are through the roof. Return to the meal plan, and make adjustments. It's simply a matter of going to and fro and plugging things in, seeing what they say, and tweaking things until you hit your macros.

If you're taking a shot at it on your own, allow me to share a few little helpful hacks. In terms of convenience, protein shakes are always the easiest way to get protein levels up. I certainly don't advocate only drinking shakes, as you should get your food from whole food sources such as chicken, pork, beef, and eggs, but for ease and convenience and price, protein shakes are great. If you can afford real, whole foods, go for it! That's awesome. But if you can't—and most of us can't—then protein shakes are an excellent choice. They're a staple part of all my clients' diets. Most people struggle eating enough protein from whole foods because most animal protein also has fat, so that might mess with meeting their fat numbers. I'll have clients say, "Adam, I ate all the meat you told me to, but it means my fats have been through the roof." It's about finding balance and then using protein shakes and protein bars as a way to make up for the difference. Most of us are inherently lazy, and that's human nature. We don't want to do all this work. If you don't want to do it, let me do it for you. I offer personal coaching services as well and would be happy to personalise your program and fast-track your results.

When you're starting out, be sure to include the

number-one thing you can't live without. I love pizza and ice cream more than most people, and that's why I don't advocate a health-guru lifestyle where you have to eat chia seeds, spinach, and kale—I don't like those kinds of foods. I always try to convince myself that pizza is healthy. It has all the food groups! It has protein on it, it has vegetables on it, and it has bread. What more do you need? I'm basically a two-hundred-kilo guy living inside a healthy guy's body. If I let myself go, I could reach two hundred kilos within a year. Knowing myself, I had to find a way where I could keep that two-hundred-kilo guy at bay and still feed him some things he enjoys from time to time to appease those binges from happening. If I went cold turkey and ate nothing but rabbit food, I would break at some point and bury myself inside an ice cream container, polishing it off in one go (I've done it before, and I will no doubt do it again—just thinking about ice cream is making me want to go and do it now!)

Most people come back with, "I'd love chocolate every day," or "I'd love pasta." It's important to work your favourite foods into your weekly meal plan at least once a week to stave off that two-hundred-kilo version of yourself wanting to binge on it every other day. I have pizza every Friday, for example. I've found ways to make pizzas less calorific but still satisfying to my taste buds. I also eat ice cream nearly every single day—watch my Snapchat story, and you will see. As part of my daily meal plans, I plug in the macros for ice cream first, and then I make everything else work around that. And because I eat ice cream every day, I rarely overeat it.

Including your favourite "unhealthy" foods in your meal plan is essential. Otherwise you'll suffer from what I call the pink elephant theory: If I tell you you're not allowed to eat chocolate, all you'll think about is chocolate. We're like children. When we were kids, if someone told us not to touch the remote, the only thing we'd think about was touching that remote. There was a Cadbury's factory close to where I live, and the chocolate company allowed its employees to eat as much chocolate as they wanted during their shift. Most employees thought it was the best thing ever, but within a week, they'd eaten themselves stupid on so much chocolate that they didn't want it anymore. If Cadbury had told its employees they were not allowed to have chocolate, I reckon every single one of them would have come up with sneaky ways to do so.

As soon as we restrict something, especially something that we enjoy, we'll end up binging on it at some point. My philosophy is about embracing the foods we know aren't the healthiest, but making it work in the meal plan.

4

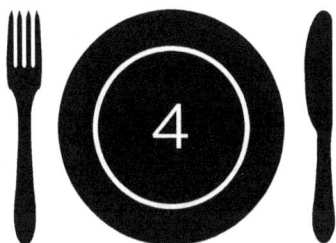

STAGE THREE: PROTEIN IS KING

Proteins are the building blocks for us to keep or build lean muscle mass. Getting in adequate protein is paramount because your body uses protein to build and repair tissues. You also use protein to make enzymes, hormones, and other body chemicals, and it's an important building block of bones, muscles, cartilage, skin, and blood. When I ask people to keep a daily diary to give me an idea of what their current diet consists of, I've time and time again found that most people eat far too many carbohydrates and fats and nowhere near enough protein. On average, from the pool of my own clients, most of them ate less than 50 percent of their daily protein minimum. And unlike fat and carbohydrates, the body does not store protein, so it doesn't have a reservoir to draw on when it needs a new supply—apart from the lean muscle we already have, and we certainly don't want to lose that!

You need protein regardless of your goals. If you do a strength-based program where you're trying to build your muscle base, you need adequate protein. If you go on a restrictive diet, trying to lose weight, you need protein to combat the loss of muscle when you do lose weight. You not only lose fat in a weight-loss program; you also lose muscle—and that's inevitable. To minimise the amount of muscle loss and maximise the amount of fat loss, you need to eat enough protein.

Say a group signs up for a weight-loss program where participants restrict their calories. They're not worrying about protein intake, and they're not doing a whole lot of strength training. They're only counting calories—calories in, calories out. You see them all the time, jogging on the treadmill or going for runs and not eating much. They might end up losing twenty or more kilos in a few months, and some think that's great, but is it? That twenty kilos isn't only fat loss; it's also muscle loss. These people may have lost ten to eleven kilos of fat, but the rest of it was muscle—and you don't want that.

Everyone talks about how your metabolism drops when

you go on a restrictive diet. While that is loosely true, they're saying it incorrectly. We've already established that muscle is an active organ within our bodies and that it needs energy. The biceps, the quads, the abs, the back—every bit of muscle we have in us needs energy to survive. If you start dropping your lean muscle mass in a weight-loss program, you start dropping the amount of calories your body needs to survive. When people say, "Oh, your metabolism drops when you go on a weight-loss program," what they're referring to is the fact that your metabolism drops because you're losing lean muscle mass. If you can maintain a lot of that lean muscle mass as you lose weight, because you're losing that weight from fat, your metabolism and the amount of calories you need each day remains about the same.

It's important to understand the concept of calories in, calories out, and that's why I stress it in stage two. If nothing else, if you get that right, you *will* lose weight. It's not going to be the best ratio of weight loss, but you'll lose weight.

My sister is a good example of a complete novice to the world of fitness. She hated going to the gym, and she hated working out—she basically hated any physical activity that wasn't walking her dog. In an effort to ease people into the program, especially for those novice people like my sister, I try not to overwhelm them with too many details, because otherwise they'd quit too early in the process. I do push increasing their protein intake, however, because it's going to become important later down the line when we introduce exercise. I created the program so each person can take his or her own pace in getting there.

If I introduced the three fundamental stages to my program up front and said, "Bob, we're going to reduce your calories, but we're going to make you eat much more protein than you've ever eaten before, and you're going to have to start doing strength training three times a week," Bob would turn to me and say, "Whoa, hang on. I can't eat the amount of protein you're telling me to eat, and you're now asking me to eat less food *and* do things I've never done before? No, thanks." It's too much.

In my program, weeks one through four focus on skipping breakfast and introducing the idea of calories in, calories out. Your macronutrient numbers are based off of your height, weight, age, and goals, and you should start tracking during this beginning stage to familiarise yourself with the foods you would eat on a day-to-day basis. Participants learn a great deal about how many calories are in their favourite foods, in addition to how many fats, carbs, and protein are in them. Tracking early offers an incredible eye-opening experience for most. Once you have tracked for a week, you'll begin to notice how close or how far you are from hitting your body's needs. You don't have to worry about hitting your macronutrients at the start of the program, but that's where we're heading, so it's good to start doing what I call "homework" so that it's not a complete surprise to you later.

Once we get to week five and I say, "Okay Bob, now you must hit that protein number," it's not something that is totally foreign to him. After tracking and familiarising himself with which of his favourite foods are loaded with protein, starting to plan his days to hit his protein number shouldn't be a brand-new thing for him. Since Bob has been tracking the daily foods he eats in his diet, he should be able to use his knowledge and plan his meals for the day in order to hit his protein count. Bob might need a couple of hundred grams of chicken a day, but he can also include some bacon because he can't live without it. To make sure he reaches his protein macros, he might need to drink a protein shake, too. During stage one, he has learned where he can get his protein from so that on day one he does not go through the shock of thinking, *Oh, my god, I need half a kilo of chicken.*

Having lean muscle makes your weight-loss journey easier because you can eat more. Let's say, as an example, a 100-kilo male has 20% body fat. That means he has 80 kilos of lean muscle mass. This person at 100 kilos who has 80 kilos of lean muscle mass is going to be completely different in regards to how much energy his body burns compared to Bob who is also 100 kilos but who has 50% body fat, meaning he only has 50 kilos of lean muscle mass.

When I give a program to John, who has 80 kilos of lean body mass, and Bob, who has 50 kilos, their meal plans and the amount of calories they can each consume on a daily basis will be vastly different. If you can increase your lean muscle mass, the amount of food you're allowed to eat as you continue to drop weight is going to be relative to the amount of lean muscle mass you have. A lot of other programs emphasise burning calories, which encourage you to hit the treadmill, go running, and eat restricted calories. Those who participate in these programs end up losing a lot of lean muscle mass. They then have to recalculate how much they can eat when they're 20 kilos lighter because they've lost muscle in addition to fat.

Say Bob, who was at 50% body fat, dropped 20 kilos, 10 of which was in muscle mass. He now has to calculate his calorie intake by 40 kilos of lean muscle mass, not 50 kilos because he lost 10 kilos of muscle. His body's lean muscle mass thus needs less energy to operate. He's already on a restrictive diet—that's how he lost the weight in the first place—and now I'll say, "Okay Bob, you lost 20 kilos. That's awesome. Now let's reduce your food even more." He'll respond, "Hang on. I'm already restricting my calories, and you want me to reduce them even more?" This is why strength training is crucial, which we'll talk about more in detail in chapter 6. Even though eating protein will help your body from losing muscle mass, the only way to build or maintain lean muscle mass is by strength training.

You cannot put on lean muscle mass by only eating protein. It has to be combined with strength training. If Bob were a personal client of mine rather than part of a program, I would have different phases that he would go through, depending on his goals. I'd say, "It's important for you to lose some weight, Bob. You're going to feel better because of it, and losing a few kilos will motivate you. Let's slam you for the next six weeks and get some weight off so you'll feel great. After that, I'm going to change things up. You're going to probably gain a little bit of weight over the following six weeks because I'm going to add some strength training. Let's build some lean muscle. You'll probably put on a few kilos, but you'll also lose fat at the same time. Weight on the scale might not change a whole lot, but you might say that your measurements around your waist go down." Once we're at that stage, we don't focus on the scale because it's a poor reflection of progress.

With my personal coaching clients, the program becomes

a much more tailored process from week to week, depending on the end goal and how much time they're willing to put into it. Clients usually hire me for five to twelve months, depending on what they want.

A lot of contestants—not all, but most—from shows like *The Biggest Loser* eventually regain all the weight they lose because there was no education surrounding eating enough protein and building lean muscle mass. Even though the show's producers make it look as if they film every week, in reality they probably film for about three weeks to produce one week's worth of content. The show claims that these people lose ten kilos in a week, but the math doesn't add up to me; it simply cannot happen. Maybe I am wrong and should give them more credit, but if one kilogram contains about 9,000 calories, and you multiply that by 10, you get 90,000 calories. This would mean the contestants need to be in a caloric deficit of more than 12,000 calories a day to lose 10 kilos in a week. In reality, the contestants are maybe eating 1,000 calories a day inside that house completely dictated by the show's hosts. It's a highly controlled environment with the amount of food they're allowed to eat, but of course for TV, they throw in some biscuits every now and then so they can catch some difficult challenges and controversy. These contestants then exercise for five to six hours a day. There's a huge discrepancy between their calories in versus calories out. They do some strength training, and you see them throwing things around mud pits and what not, but that's a bit of theater because it's better to see a guy crawling through the dirt than bench-pressing some weights at the gym. In the eyes of major TV networks, weight lifting is boring to watch. I certainly don't think it's boring, as I love that sort of thing (if you do, too, and want some motivation, I highly recommend watching the show on Netflix called *Froning*. It's fair to say I have a man crush on Matt Froning, the protagonist in the show, as he attempts to win big at the CrossFit Games). A lot of the exercises these *Biggest Loser* contestants do are high-intensity-based cardio. They're spending hours upon hours on treadmills, steppers, and cross-trainers, and from my observation in watching the show, there isn't a whole lot of macro planning.

I have no problem giving these contestants credit when credit is due. They still lose a bucket load of weight, but a lot of that weight is muscle mass. If Susie is named the biggest loser after the show is over, the world will be in awe of her incredible results. "Congratulations, Susie! You are 50 percent of your starting body weight!" She then returns to the real world where she's immediately surrounded by food again. She quickly realises her journey on the show didn't help her change her bad habits, nor was she educated about how to keep the weight off or to even sustainably maintain her new weight. She likely lost so much lean muscle mass during her time on the show that her metabolism (the amount of calories her body needs to function) is now much lower than what it could've been if the show's hosts had her lift weights and eat more protein. Even eating what would be considered a standard calorie intake is likely more than what her body needs after the show, and it's no wonder most contestants regain most, if not all, of their weight.

The same goes for anyone crash-dieting in the absence of strength training. You reach this fantastic weight you've always been hoping for and then think, *Great! I made it to my goal weight, so now I'll eat maintenance calories.* Your real maintenance calories, however, are much, much lower now. You start eating what you think is fine for you, when in reality it's too much, and you inevitably gain weight again.

I have watched shows inviting previous *Biggest Loser* contestants to discuss what happened after the show, revealing that most contestants gained all their weight back. One of our current affair shows in Australia gathered up many of the contestants over the last six or seven seasons to update the world on what happened to them once the show aired. Turns out, a large portion of the contestants who lost weight were now heavier or at least the same weight they were before they appeared on the show. And of course these contestants all had a sob story, which I admit might be a little theater to put on TV—but a lot of them were struggling. They all seemed to say that they hadn't learned anything. They were drilled to the point of exhaustion every day and then told, "Here's your cupboard worth of food. That's all you're getting." After the show, when they returned home and real life hadn't changed, they returned to their old habits.

I find those stories extremely sad, and I don't want to see that happen to you.

EATING ENOUGH PROTEIN

A lot of people struggle in eating the amount of protein their body needs. There's no magic pill for it, either. Set a goal, and slowly build to where you need to be. As stated in the last chapter, to figure out your optimal amount of protein, multiply your weight in pounds by 0.6 to 1. If you are a 160-pound woman, you should aim to eat between 96 and 150 grams of protein every day. If you're a 200-pound man, you should aim to eat 120 to 200 grams.

When I set people's macronutrients and tell them they need 100 grams of protein a day, they sometimes misunderstand that to mean they need 100 grams of chicken.

This is wrong. We are measuring the amount of the macronutrient protein in chicken, not the weight of the chicken itself. Chicken is not only made of protein. In 100 grams of chicken, for example, there are only 25 grams of protein. Protein can also be found in eggs, dairy, cheese, and beans. A lot of protein is in steak, chicken, eggs, and all the different kind of animal products we have. You can also find protein in chickpeas, nuts, and peanut butter. Be careful, however, because most foods have more than one macronutrient, so the challenge is to eat enough protein without going over with the other macronutrients.

You might think nuts are a good source of protein, but truth be told, they're not, because they're loaded with fat. One hundred grams of nuts have around 25 grams of protein; 100 grams of steak also has 25 grams of protein.

This might make you think, *Nuts are as good as steak.* On the surface, sure, both items have the same amount of protein, but the nuts also have 50 grams of fat, meaning there are around 600 calories in 100 grams of nuts; whereas 100 grams of steak only have 200 calories—that's a big difference.

Balancing your macros and reaching the level of protein is hard, but have no fear! That's why we have protein powders and protein bars. In a perfect world, it'd be great

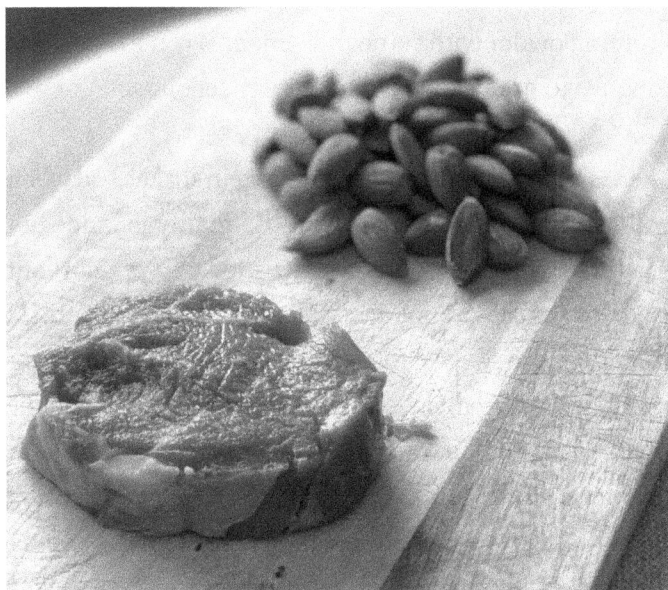

to nail our macros from whole foods like animal products, eggs, and dairy. In the real world, however, it can be quite difficult—and it's not cheap, either. Buying steak is expensive. Even yoghurt is expensive (the ones that aren't overloaded with sugar). Most protein powders, on the other hand, are quite affordable. They're roughly a dollar per serving—and there are some out there that are even less than that. Eating between 100 and 180 grams of protein every day is a lot, so I use protein powder daily. If you tried to eat that many grams of protein naturally, you would have to eat half a kilo of chicken—every day!—and that's a lot of chewing. After a while, you'll get to a point where you say, "Ugh. Not this again." Mixing a scoop of protein powder with some milk enables you to consume roughly 30 grams of protein in thirty seconds.

There's a lot of marketing around protein shakes and when you should consume them, but the reality is it doesn't matter. You'll see products claim they're a preworkout drink or a postworkout drink, but there's not a whole lot of evidence to suggest that timing is that important, especially for the normal person trying to lose some weight. If you're an athlete training for the Olympics, then sure, there are some definite benefits to timing your eating window. But for you, for me, for 98 percent of the population, it doesn't matter when you drink your protein shakes.

What's more important is finding one that tastes good to you because, unfortunately, there are a lot that taste horrible. It's also important to find one that's 75–80 percent protein per 100 grams. Protein powders that fall into this range usually have marginal fats and carbohydrates associated with them. Watch out for those that taste absolutely divine, too. If they taste like real chocolate ice cream, it's probably because they have heaps of sugar in them, which of course means they probably have a lot of carbohydrates. There's certainly nothing wrong with that, but some people might want to save those carbs for something else. In the end it's up to you and what you can work with. For me personally, I'd rather drink one that is pure protein with low carbs so I can enjoy ice cream that same day.

Most later-day eaters have two meals a day with some snacks. They'll have their first meal around lunchtime, followed by an afternoon snack, then dinner and possibly some postdinner snacks. If we can make it fit your day, you might have some sort of dessert in there as well. If you're someone who likes to have meals every few hours, then that's what you should do. If you prefer big meals and you're happy to sacrifice smaller meals elsewhere to have that big meal, then that's what you should do.

To help with increasing your protein intake, start incorporating some protein at every meal. Say it's lunch, for example, and you usually enjoy a sandwich with a single slice of ham and salad. You're not eating a big heap of protein, so I'd suggest you include more slices of ham, or perhaps even add turkey to increase flavour and protein. I would also look at the salad and make sure there's a hard-boiled egg, some chicken breast, or even some quinoa to boost up the protein.

PRIMARY SOURCES OF PROTEIN

Seafood: Seafood is an excellent source of protein because it's usually low in fat. Fish such as salmon is a little higher in fat, so be careful; however, it does contain omega-3 fatty acids, which can be good for your heart. But remember, calories in must equal calories out.

White-meat poultry: Stick to the white meat of poultry for excellent, lean protein. Dark meat is a little higher in fat. The skin is loaded with fat, so remove the skin before cooking. If you'd like to impart some delicious flavour from the skin, leave it on while cooking it, and then take it off before eating.

Milk, cheese, and yoghurt: Not only are dairy foods like milk, cheese, and yoghurt excellent sources of protein, but they also contain valuable calcium, and many are fortified with vitamin D. Just be mindful, as foods like cheese are extremely high in fat and can be hard to fit into a day-to-day weight-loss program.

Eggs: Eggs are one of the least expensive forms of protein. Whole eggs also carry a hefty fat content, so I recommend eating egg whites to maximise the protein intake. With various companies producing cartons of only egg whites, it's a great way to get high protein and no fat without having to do it yourself, wasting all those egg yolks.

Beans: One-half cup of beans contains as much protein as thirty grams of grilled steak. Plus, these nutritious nuggets are loaded with fibre to keep you feeling full for hours.

Pork tenderloin: This great and versatile white meat is 31 percent leaner than it was twenty years ago.

Soy: Eating soy protein instead of sources of higher-fat protein can be good for your heart.

Lean beef: It has only one more gram of saturated fat than a skinless chicken breast and is also an excellent source of zinc, iron, and vitamin B12.

VEGETARIANS AND VEGANS

Vegetarians and vegans will certainly find eating enough protein quite challenging, but it's definitely possible. It's a lot easier now than it was ten years ago. There are protein powders and bars that are vegan or vegetarian friendly. Products like pea powders are also starting to become more and more accessible for those who follow a vegetarian or vegan lifestyle. It'll take a lot more planning, but it's definitely something that can be done. Take a look at Frank Medrano to see how you can live a strict vegan life and still sport a ripped physique.

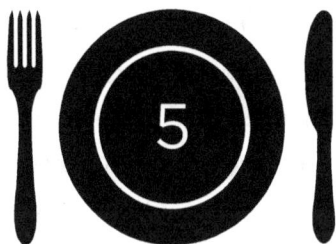

STAGE FOUR: A CARB IS A CARB AND FAT IS FAT—AT FIRST

In the beginning, it doesn't matter where you're getting your carbs or fats. A carb is a carb whether it comes from chocolate or from fruit, and a fat is a fat whether it comes from avocado or butter.

The beauty of Start Late, Stay Light is you can still eat your favourite foods. Just hit those numbers however you want to hit them, and if you hit them daily, you'll lose weight. This is why I ask what your favourite foods are from the start. The carbs you find in chocolate, for example, come from pure sugar. Most people who look at me would say

I'm in great physical shape, yet I enjoy ice cream most days of the week. I eat two or three servings of fruit and a huge serving of vegetables each day. If I'm hitting all my micronutrient needs and have some excess carbs left over, I'd rather use them on things I enjoy rather than eating more fruit or vegetables. I reckon most people would choose chocolate ice cream over a banana any day of the week.

Make the food you enjoy fit your macros. You still have to hit your protein, you still have to keep under your set calories, and you should be getting in good amounts of micronutrients from fresh fruits and fresh veggies, but once you've hit all those for the day, if you have some macros left over and you can make a little bowl of ice cream or a row of chocolate fit, do it. You can't eat the whole block of chocolate, though. You still have to be disciplined, work out how much you are allowed, and enjoy your little treat.

It's through the tracking process that you will learn what macros are in your favourite foods. I don't want you to blindly eat them and say, "Well, I know pizza is pretty high in carbs." How many carbs, exactly? If I eat ice cream, I know that's mostly carbohydrates and a bit of fat, but how many carbs and fats, exactly? Most people have no idea how many calories are in our food, and we are horrible guessers. Most people underestimate the amount of calories in our food—by a lot. By encouraging people to plug in the numbers to apps like MyFitnessPal and play around with structuring their daily meal plans, I have found that they will quickly learn the truth of what is in their food.

My Start Late, Stay Light lifestyle is truly a flexible way of eating for the rest of your life without sacrificing the foods you love. It's about planning each day and making positive food decisions that your body will benefit from. In the future, if you are going out to dinner to your favourite French restaurant and your mouth waters thinking about the restaurant's famous crème brûlée, you can plan your day from the get-go and avoid foods with a lot of carbs and fats so you can cash them in with dessert at the restaurant. With enough practise, and the help from this book, you should be able to interplay between high-fat foods, high-carb foods, and high-protein foods, and intuitively be able to do this for the rest of your life.

At this point in the program, you should already know how many carbs and fats your body needs to run like a well-oiled machine. We established those numbers in chapter 3. You have your protein set based off of your weight, 25-30 percent of your calorie intake should be in fat, and the rest goes to carbs.

WHAT YOU NEED TO KNOW ABOUT CARBS

Most of us have no problem eating enough carbs. Carbohydrates are purely used for energy, so if you're an inactive person, you don't need a lot of carbs because your body won't use it as energy and instead store it as fat. Carbohydrates are in a whole host of foods—breads, pastas, vegetables, fruits, chocolate, and of course your favourite gin and tonic—and our bodies use carbs as a fuel source. When you consume carbs, your pancreas releases insulin, and your body converts that glucose into energy. Whatever glucose isn't used up as energy is stored as fat. Look at carbs as your petrol tank. Whatever energy you need, that's where it's coming from.

THE RELATIONSHIP BETWEEN CARBS AND FIBRE

Most of the foods with fibre also have carbs. Fibre is important for our digestion and our gut health, helping with the movement of our bowels. Fibre is mostly found in our green leafy vegetables and grains. Muesli is quite high in fibre, for example. There's usually a bit of fibre in bread as long as it's whole grain. Health companies love to market that white bread is the enemy. You won't consume any fibre from white bread, but that doesn't mean it's the enemy; there are a lot of other ways you can get fibre. If you love white bread and you're eating plenty of green leafy vegetables and grains elsewhere, then I say you should enjoy your white bread. I love a fresh slice of bread straight from the bakery with a light layer of Vegemite on it—yum!

Fibre is important for our digestion and gut health, and good digestion helps alleviate colon cancer. Colon cancer is one of the most common cancers—and one of the most preventable if precancerous polyps are found early. But like other forms of cancer, colon cancer can be deadly if it isn't detected until the later stages. Colon cancer is becoming a much more prevalent cancer than a lot of people give it credit for. A diet high in fruits and vegetables appears to reduce the risk of colon cancer by about half, so be sure to include cruciferous vegetables such as cabbage, broccoli, cauliflower, and Brussels sprouts in your diet. A large study published in 2007 found that people who ate a high-fibre, low-fat diet had the same amount of colorectal adenomas (small tumors that can sometimes turn into cancer) as those who didn't eat that way. Yet when researchers from the Ohio State University Comprehensive Cancer Center zeroed in on study participants who stuck to the diet, as opposed to those who were less consistent, they did find a link between eating lots of fibre and fewer tumors.

Good sources of fibre come from beans (think three-bean

salad, bean burritos, chili, soup); whole grains (whole-wheat bread, pasta, etc.); brown rice (white rice doesn't offer much fibre); popcorn (great source of fibre); nuts (almonds, pecans, and walnuts have more fibre than other nuts); baked potato with skin (the skin is what's important here); berries (all those seeds, plus the skin, give great fibre to any berry); bran cereal (any cereal that has five grams of fibre or more in a serving counts as high fibre); oatmeal (whether its microwaved or stove-cooked, oatmeal is good fibre); and vegetables (the crunchier, the better).

Just like there are protein bars, there are also various supplemental products that focus on fibre. Fibre One bars and Quest Bars are well-known brands, for example. Some products are manufactured fibre that you can stir in water and drink—like Metamucil. Fibre supplements come in many forms, from capsules to powders to chewable tablets. They contain what's called "functional fibre," which may be extracted from natural sources or made in a lab. They'll certainly help with getting your fibre content up, but I would still encourage consuming it from natural sources. Taking supplements won't make up for poor eating habits. You can't take an unhealthy diet and put in supplements and think that it all of the sudden becomes a healthy diet.

When it comes to fibre bars, watch out for the amount of carbs and fats. Quest Bars are high in fibre, and the company promotes its bars as only having five grams of carbs, when in reality, there's more. In small brackets, you'll see something called "net carbs" because the bars also contain 25 grams of carbs. Fibre is a different form of carb, but at the end of the day, it's still a carb. Quest Bars and Fibre One bars taste great and can be an easy way to help meet your daily fibre goals, but they can also be expensive.

Don't overdo it on the fibre supplements, either; it *is* possible to consume too much fibre. Studies suggest that adding fifty or more grams per day may affect how your body absorbs nutrients, so be sure to think about how much fibre you consume overall, from both diet and supplements, when figuring out how much you need.

SUGAR IS A CARB

People eat far too much sugar in general. For longevity, if people can make it work in their diet, great! I'm a walking example of that since I eat ice cream every single day. I also visit the doctor for annual checkups to make sure I'm as healthy on the inside as I look on the outside. I have my blood tested to make sure my resting blood glucose (so I'm not at risk of type two diabetes) and my cholesterol (so I'm not at risk of heart disease) are normal. I implore you to see a doctor annually, especially males because we never do it.

Glucose is the primary source of energy your body uses, and every cell relies on it to function. When we talk about blood sugar, we are referring to glucose in the blood.

Fructose, or fruit sugar, is a simple sugar naturally occurring in fruit, honey, sucrose, and high-fructose corn syrup. Fructose is super sweet, roughly one and a half times sweeter than sucrose (white sugar). Because of the worldwide increase in the consumption of sweeteners, soft drinks, and foods containing high-fructose corn syrup, fructose intake has quadrupled since the early 1900s.

Sucrose is crystallised white sugar produced by the sugarcane plant and can be found in households and foods worldwide. Sucrose is a disaccharide made up of 50 percent glucose and 50 percent fructose and is broken down rapidly into its constituent parts.

Lactose is a sugar found in milk. It is a disaccharide made up of glucose and galactose units. It is broken down into the two parts by an enzyme called lactase. Once broken down, the simple sugars can be absorbed into the bloodstream.

Anything that ends in "-ose" is basically a broken-down form of the food that we're eating and what it turns into so our bodies can metabolise it. It's all still sugar, whether it comes from a banana or a glass of milk. No matter the food source, once the body breaks it down, the body still sees it as a sugar.

Bottom line: There are two types of sugar—naturally occurring sugar such as lactose in milk, and added sugar, which includes table sugar (sucrose) as well as concentrated sources such as fruit juice.

WHAT YOU NEED TO KNOW ABOUT FATS

Fats have had a bad rap for years now, but in reality, this misunderstood macronutrient provides a wealth of health benefits. Fats are energy rich, containing nine calories per gram—more than twice the amount in carbohydrates and protein. Stored throughout the body, as well as the liver and muscles, fat serves as a large energy reserve that can be tapped into at rest or during low-intensity exercise. In addition, vitamins A, D, E, and K are fat-soluble vitamins, so without adequate fat, these vitamins couldn't be absorbed, transported, or used in the body, resulting in various deficiencies.

Unfortunately, fats are still battling their bad reputation.

We can look as far back as the 1970s when governments first told us to follow low-fat diets and minimise saturated fats to reduce the risk of cardiovascular disease, cancer, high blood pressure, and everything in between. What followed was a monumental shift in the food industry toward promoting low-fat foods, slapping low-fat claims on any and every food item in sight.

The thought process looked something like this: "Cholesterol is coming from animal products. Animal products have fat in them, therefore we should stop eating fat." That's when all of those fat-free muffins, fat-free ice cream, and fat-free chocolates started coming out, claiming, "See? We don't have any fat anymore! Now we're all good again!" Unfortunately, this has bred a false mentality among a lot of people who think buying fat-free yoghurt is healthy. "I'm having fat-free yoghurt; therefore, I can have the entire tub, and I'm completely fine." Wrong. It might be fat-free, but that doesn't mean it's calorie-free. Also, if you take fat out of something, it becomes an unstable product, so you have to add something back in it to make it stable again—and that something is usually some sort of sugar or vegetable gum stabiliser. These additives, though nasty, are basically just high in sugar—simple carbohydrates—so if they aren't used, our bodies immediately store the energy as fat.

People have this idea that if it's fat-free, it's good for me, which is not the case. You can't walk down a shopping aisle without seeing 80 percent of products saying fat-free on them, and they're usually in a green package as well because green means health, right? Marketers are clever at making you think that a product is good for you if it says "all natural" or if it's in a green packet—and then you think you can have three of these bars every night. That's not the case.

Having said all that, I do eat fat-free yoghurt because I save my fats for the ice cream I eat every night (have I mentioned how much I love ice cream?). I'm constantly interplaying where I get my fats, and I'm usually getting them from sources I find more enjoyable. I have nothing against eating fat-free products, but you need to understand that fat-free doesn't mean you can eat as much of it as you'd like.

BREAKING DOWN SOME FATS

The fats we ingest with our food contain both saturated and unsaturated fatty acids. Saturated fatty acids can be mainly found in animal foods such as butter, cream, and cheese, but also in some vegetable fats such as palm or coconut oil. These fatty acids are also referred to as "unhealthy" fats. Monounsaturated fatty acids are contained in mostly vegetable oils such as olive and rapeseed oil. Polyunsaturated fatty acids are vital for our bodies, as we can't produce them ourselves. Here, a distinction is made between omega-6 fatty acids (contained in sunflower, corn, and soy oil) and omega-3 fatty acids (found in herring, salmon, mackerel, nuts, or seeds). Omega-3 fatty acids protect the cardiovascular system while preventing coronary diseases. Moreover, they positively affect our cholesterol levels by raising the so-called good cholesterol (HDL) and also play a vital role in brain development. You want to try and stay clear of trans fats. I won't go into the nitty-gritty behind why they're so bad, but understand that they are the Darth Vader of fats, if you will, and you want to avoid them as much as possible.

If you're in a healthy weight range and your cholesterol is fine, your blood pressure is fine, and you'd rather get your fats from a saturated fat—an animal fat instead of an unsaturated fat such as olive oil—then I say go for it. Visit your doctor, check yourself every year, and if you're in a healthy weight range and your blood work falls into healthy ranges, then keep doing what you're doing. If you're in the bad ranges, you need to make a change.

TRUST THE PROCESS

By now, you should have a good understanding of calories

in, calories out and the three macronutrients: protein, carbs, and fats. You should know what your macros are, and you should be tracking your food and hitting your macro numbers consistently.

This is the stage, five to eight weeks into Start Late, Stay Light, where people start to flounder. This is natural and part of the process. The beginning was relatively easy, and you might have lost some weight. Week three came and went, and you might have fallen off the wagon a little bit, but you still saw some weight loss. Week four approached, and your friend might have thrown a birthday party where you ate a slice of chocolate cake and didn't track it. We all have ups and downs—no one is perfect. Then week five comes and you might fall off track a little bit more, reverting back to old habits. Are you getting enough protein? It all might be a bit much, and you stop seeing progress, so you think, *Well, this program doesn't work, because I didn't lose weight two weeks in a row*, but you've forgotten about that cake you ate three times last week. We're all good at convincing ourselves we did everything right and acted like angels when it comes to nutrition.

At this stage, like in any program, it becomes a bit overwhelming because it's finally settling in that this is a daily grind, it's day in and day out, and it's hard work. It's not easy; it's simple to do, but it's not easy to implement.

Naturally, my sister hit a stage where she struggled as well. Because she had quite a bit of weight to lose, she spent a little more time with each stage and therefore didn't hit her plateau until later. She lost weight consistently for a good ten weeks before it started to slow down, and that's when she started thinking negatively and doubting the program's continual success. She called me and said, "I did everything you taught me," and I believed her. She tracked her food, didn't start eating until the afternoon, followed her meal plan, and drank plenty of water. Between her ten- and twelve-week mark, she didn't see much progress on the scale, which can be discouraging—I understand that. She was hyperfocused on that scale at that time, and when she didn't see any weight loss, she interpreted that as failure.

"Hang on," I said to her. "We're at ten weeks, and you've lost ten kilos. You're telling me you're a failure?"

It happens to all of us. We enter dark thoughts and beat ourselves up for everything, sometimes forgetting all the work we've put in up until that moment.

My sister is a teacher, and when she hit this plateau between ten and twelve weeks, it also coincided with an incredibly busy time at work. "I had so many reports to write," she would say. "I came home late, and I didn't have time to work out." I said, "Full respect, I understand that, but you have to remember why you're doing this and fully commit." I pushed her to keep at it and reminded her how working out on those days when we think we don't have time are the most important days to work out. She pushed through, elevated her level of commitment, and when she reached twenty-six weeks, she was twenty-seven kilos lighter. She kept pushing forward, and she now trusts the program because she's been through tough times and came out better on the other side of it. No doubt, there will be another tough time—perhaps quite a few—and as they come, she'll know to power through them because she's done it before.

Whenever you hit these moments of frustration, doubt, or plateaus, you have to remember why you started this program five to six weeks ago. Return to your "why." It's because you want to be healthy and fit for your kids. It's because you want to be a good role model for them. It's because you want to look good in a bikini or squeeze into that wedding dress. Whatever it might be, return to your "why," and be honest with yourself. Have you been sticking to it? If you haven't, what have you been doing? Identify your pitfalls. How can you do better? Don't look at anything as good or bad—it's not about defining your actions as good or bad. Instead, identify areas that need improvement, where you can make correct choices to continually improve your fitness and continue your weight loss. Remember, fitness is a never-ending science experiment that you are conducting on yourself to figure out what works for you and what doesn't.

Progress is not a straight line. You will have victories, and you will have setbacks; it's not an exponential process. You don't lose weight every single day. There are times (especially for females when you're going through your menstrual cycle) when your weight will go up; it'll happen. Our bodies are always fighting us to not lose weight because of the way our bodies are programmed. Our bodies hate losing weight, and your body will fight you every step of the way, even when you get to the stage that is considered healthy and fit.

Fitness is a daily grind for me, too. Watch my Snapchat, and you will see that I struggle like everyone else. It takes dedication and commitment, and it's not easy. It's not like once you reach your goal weight, you can go back to what you were doing before. It doesn't mean you stop exercising and stop tracking. This lifestyle is day in, day out, and that thought can overwhelm people: "Oh, my god. This is for the next sixty years of my life!" That can be a tough thought to wrap your head around.

You can either accept that fact, keep pushing, and keep

working hard at it, or not accept it and return to your old ways and gain weight again. It's as simple as that. You can sit there and complain to me all day that you have the hardest life in the world, that you work eighty hours a week and have three children. Your life might be rough, sure, but if you want to change your health and live a happier, healthier, and longer life, then sorry! I'm not going to accept your excuses. Put up, shut up, and do the work. What's your priority? If your priorities lie with sitting on the couch and watching *Game of Thrones*, then fine. There's nothing wrong with that, but you can't then turn around and complain to me that the program doesn't work because you're not losing weight and you're not where you want to be. That's your fault, not mine. The program works if you stick to it and do it—and you can do it! There will be tough times along the way, but you'll reach your goals if you have patience and keep working. I do not accept lack of time as an excuse, either; we all have busy lives. Health should always be a top priority because, in my opinion, if you don't have health, you have nothing.

"The pain of self-discipline is better than the pain of regret." I love this quotation, and my clients will testify to how often I use it. It's hard to be self-disciplined every single day—trust me, I know; I struggle with it, too. Mustering the energy to go for a run at 7:00 p.m. at night when you normally did it at 5:00 p.m. is an uphill battle; you don't feel like getting off the couch. We all have these moments, and it's hard as hell to motivate ourselves. But in the end, that's a hell of a lot easier than the pain and regret you're going to feel the next day when you're kicking yourself, saying, "God, I wish I ran, because now I've fallen off a little bit, and now I'm going backward rather than moving forward." Or even worse, imagine how you will feel when you are on that hospital bed after having a massive heart attack, thinking about how you could have taken better care of yourself. If you want to live a long and healthy life to cherish with your kids, then health better be your number-one priority. Stop telling me you don't have time, because we all have enough time—it's a matter of how we choose to spend it. "Not having time" is a bullshit excuse.

Allow me to let you in on a little secret: There will never be a time that's easier than right now. People always say, "I'll start my diet on Monday," or, "I'll start that running program on Monday." It's always either a New Year's resolution or something to start on the first of the month. Why is the first of January any different than the fourteenth of December? It's exactly the same twenty-four hours, so start now. Start today! Why postpone it? Focus on the now.

Trust the process. Trust in me that I do have your best interest at heart and that this process works and you will succeed. If you practise enough patience and you put in the work, you'll succeed. The first time people hit a major setback (because they've been let down on so many other programs) is usually when they succumb to defeat and say, "See? It doesn't work for me. I'm one of those people who never loses weight." Well, no, we're all the same; keep pushing through it. If you're honest throughout these moments, and you know they're an inevitable part of the process, you can mentally prepare yourself to deal with them. These moments also can signify a need to change course and be honest with yourself, like admitting you ate chocolate cake at a party.

This lifestyle will set you up for the rest of your life, and you'll live that happier, healthier, and longer life so you can spend it with your family. And that in itself, in my opinion, is totally worth it.

6

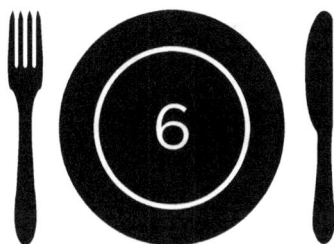

STAGE FIVE: MOVEMENT

Exercise is important for continued weight loss because it builds and maintains lean muscle mass. The biggest mistake many people make with regards to exercise as part of a weight-loss journey is focusing more on performing cardiovascular activities rather than strength training. They think that if they burn more calories via cardio exercise than they're eating, the number on the scale will move in their favor. While that is correct on the surface—a super macro surface—cardio exercises, whether working on a cross-trainer for two hours or going for a run, don't have the same effect on your lean muscle tissue as strength training does, be it building it or maintaining it. As previously mentioned, strength training is hugely important in weight loss because it'll maintain your lean muscle mass. While cardio-type exercises are important for a lot of other reasons (we'll get to that shortly), they should be viewed as a tool to help you along your journey; they're certainly not the golden ticket to lose weight.

Your main focus should be to build more muscle. If you've led a pretty active life and are satisfied with where you're at, you might be looking to maintain what you have. But if you're looking to lose weight and sculpt a healthy body, lifting heavy objects is the way to go, one hundred percent.

"But I'm a beginner and have never even seen a dumbbell before, Adam! I'm scared!" For beginners especially, strength training should be your main focus. Let's take Susie, who's never stepped inside the gym before. She's thirty kilos overweight—weight that has crept on over time—but she takes frequent walks with her girlfriend and has two kids she runs around with every day. It's the typical scenario where weight creeps up over the years but not enough to motivate the individual to buckle down and start paying for a gym membership. These newbies respond well to strength training in the beginning because they've never built muscle before. Lifting heavy objects essentially shocks their bodies, and they therefore react quickly to the new stimulation. After a few weeks, Susie could build a bit of strength and muscle while also starting the process of losing fat.

Then there's Bob, who may have been a high-level athlete when he was younger. He's been to the gym before and is familiar with lifting weights, but maybe work derailed his gym time over the last few years. He's also a father and has kept busy with kids, despite his travel schedule. His response to strength training will be a bit slower compared to a full-on beginner because his body's much more accustomed to it. He's definitely in a better place in terms of lean muscle mass because he's done it before, and he certainly has a different level of fitness, but seeing results compared to Susie will take a bit longer. His goal therefore might be more focused on maintaining what he has while he drops some weight, whereas Susie could put on a little bit of lean muscle mass and lose fat at the same time.

Unfortunately, the gym can be counterproductive to weight loss for some. There are quite a lot of studies that have found that people who exercise tend to eat more. Yes, I know what you might be thinking. "Well, duh! Of course they're going to eat more; they're burning more calories." The problem comes in our justification of fulfilling our *wants* as opposed to focusing on what our bodies *need*. Come evening time when you have finished your day of eating with what your bodies *needs*, you still justify your *wants* by saying, "I did a gym workout today. What's an extra cookie?" or, "What's an extra piece of fruit?" Whatever the food may be, we are good at rewarding ourselves with eating more. "I worked out today, so that means I can have it." We're programmed to match our energy-in and energy-out levels; in other words, our brain will always say, "Well, you expended 300 calories; I need that back." Most of us eat more than what the brain is telling us because we're not actually listening to it. We say, "I want that cake," or, "I want that glass of wine." It comes from a place of I *want* rather than I *need*.

So how do we circumvent this overindulging behavior? We plan our meals out. When we engage in cardio exercises, we usually do it for a half hour or an hour, which would burn 600 to 700 calories at the top end—and I mean the tippy-top end as it is more likely to be around the 350 to 500 mark for most people. One chocolate bar can completely neutralise this. Planning is the key to avoid overeating and neutralising your exercise. Plan your meals for each week, and stick to them. Incorporate your favourite foods, like pizza or ice cream, to avoid overindulging, and keep hitting your macros for the day. Maybe one day you plan to eat a burger for lunch, some fruit in the afternoon, and then a salad at night. If something wasn't a part of your plan for the day, you're less likely to overeat, so follow your meal plan!

A TOOL FOR WEIGHT LOSS

Exercise is a tool for weight loss, not the route to weight loss. Nutrition always trumps exercise. We've all heard the saying, "Weight loss is 90 percent nutrition, 10 percent exercise," or "You can't outrun a bad diet." Well, it's true. Exercise is a great tool to even out excess calories on those days we overindulge, but you can't eat horribly, run every day, and expect to be a fitness model. Cardiovascular exercise is purely a tool in helping with energy balance. It can certainly quicken weight loss when we need a jump start, but these tactics need to be conducted in a specific circumstance, because over the long-term, they are simply not sustainable. I'll share an example.

When my sister first started this program, she made a goal. She planned a trip of a lifetime to Europe for four weeks, and her goal was to lose twenty-seven kilos before leaving. She had twenty-six weeks. She adopted the Start Late, Stay Light lifestyle and saw amazing progress from week one. Four days before boarding that plane, she stepped on the scale, and it was twenty-six kilos down from her starting weight. She was determined, though, so in order to reach her goal, we looked to drastic measures. I would never suggest this as part of any normal program, but in order for her to drop that final kilo, I put her on a heavy cardio regimen. We boosted as much energy expenditure as we could in those four days, and she increased her cardio time to three hours. She kept her protein level the same to maintain her lean muscle mass, but I told her to avoid carbs. She didn't eat any carbohydrates for those four days. This strategy allowed her to shed a heap of water weight through sweating and not consuming any carbohydrates, since they hang on to water.

The day she was scheduled to fly to Europe, she stepped on the scale, and she did it! BOOM! In four days, she dropped 1.7 kilos. These are the kinds of things I do as little hacks sometimes if people are feeling a little down, defeated, or ready to quit, because it offers a bit of a jolt to get them excited again. That being said, it is by no means a sustainable strategy to lose a bunch of weight, and I highly discourage you from doing it for long periods of time. When people start wavering in the program, maybe because they have cheated a few times and they're not seeing any results, I'll sometimes throw these short-term hacks to show a result in order to spurt them back into it again.

BUILDING LEAN MUSCLE MASS

You might have heard that restricting your calories reduces your metabolism, but that is wrong, and I do not subscribe to it whatsoever. It all comes down to the amount of lean muscle mass you have and how much energy it needs to survive. In my program, I do ask what your body weight is purely because I want to know your starting point, but the main number that's more important is your body fat percentage because that tells me what your lean muscle mass is.

As we know, muscles require energy to exist. Each pound of muscle expends 30–60 calories per day, even if you don't use it for exercise. When you are sleeping, your muscles continue to use energy and burn calories. Your muscles are energy factories for you to move, and they require energy to perform their duties. The brain also uses a heap of energy to keep us ticking. Your heart, your lungs, all of your internal organs, and your muscles consume energy to function. Fat that sits around our glutes, thighs, hips, or stomach, on the other hand, is an innate object; it doesn't do much of anything. It sits there and doesn't need any energy. On the surface, it's wasted space making you heavy, whereas muscle has a function. It's the engine that sits inside your car. When you fill your car up with petrol, that's like when you feed your mouth with food.

Every muscle in your body requires energy to be alive, and we've already established the correlation between lean muscle mass and its affect on energy in, energy out; and that's why I believe strength training is the most important form of exercise.

I'd also like to point out that muscle does not weigh more than fat. That's a complete myth. If I have a kilo of muscle and a kilo of fat, it's the same as if I had a kilo of bricks and a kilo of feathers. A kilo is a kilo—you'd just need way more feathers to make a kilo compared to bricks. In the same way, you need more muscle to make a kilo compared to fat. That's why scales are a good example of long-term progress, not good for daily or weekly use, because they don't accurately portray progress.

PUTTING IT TOGETHER

You can do all the strength training in the world, but if you don't have adequate protein to fuel the workout, then you won't put on as much lean muscle mass as you could have if you'd eaten adequate protein. This is the stage where I introduce mandatory strength training, be it in the gym with weights or with body weight.

It's better to eat 100 grams of protein and build the rest of your lean muscle mass through strength training than eat 180 grams of protein and not do strength training at all. That's like building a fire with a thousand pieces of wood but no match. You could build the biggest teepee of wood, get all the kindling, and even throw some kerosene on the pile, but it won't lite itself. All it needs is a match, and it would explode. That's what weight lifting is. You can stack your body full of protein every single day, but unless you actually do something with it, nothing's going to happen. I would rather someone be a little under their protein numbers but be doing strength training than getting all the protein in the world and saying, "I just have to sit back and watch my biceps grow because Adam told me I have to eat protein." It doesn't work that way.

NOT JUST FOR BODYBUILDERS

Strength training is an integral part of a well-rounded exercise program, and it is recommended for both sexes of all ages, including kids and seniors. Building muscle through resistance exercises has many benefits, from losing excess fat to maintaining healthy bone mass and preventing age-related muscle loss as we grow older. Strength training has been demonised as being only for bodybuilders, but that couldn't be further from the truth. I think it has been demonised far too long as something for men who want big biceps to show off to girls, but it's so much more than that.

Many ignore strength training when devising their exercise plan because they don't want to "bulk up." I'd like to put to rest any worries that strength training will make you look like Arnold Schwarzenegger right now. It won't happen. Your genes and food intake control your muscle growth, and only a few have the potential to become muscle bound. The size of your muscles are also limited by your age, gender, body type, and many other biological and genetic factors. Proper strength training will increase the strength and endurance of your muscles, which will improve your cardiovascular efficiency and burn more calories and fat in the process.

In a study published in the *American Journal of Medicine*, UCLA researchers found that people with greater muscle-mass percentages lived longer than those who had less muscle. In addition to fasting, the fountain of youth can be found somewhere between the dumbbells and the pull-up bar! These findings add to a growing pile of evidence that overall body composition is a better predictor of all-cause mortality than overall weight or body mass index (BMI). I love this study because it demonstrates the importance of muscle mass in overall life expectancy and highlights the necessity to look beyond what you see in the mirror.

Bottom line: Having more lean muscle mass and being fit means you'll live longer because you'll be healthier. No one wants to lose his or her strength or ability to function independently. Muscle loss happens gradually, so you probably won't notice it occurring at first. Not only does lifting weights help you feel stronger and healthier; it can give you the ability to shovel snow on your own, carry your groceries, and pick up your grandchildren. Sure, you can reach ninety years of age through medication, but you're going to be miserable for the last fifteen years because you can't stand up, you'll be in a nursing home, and a nurse will have to shower you because you can't do it yourself.

HOW WE BUILD MUSCLE

Let's use bench presses as an example. When you bench-press, you're basically creating little, little tears in your chest muscles. The body responds by relaying micro amounts of muscle to essentially repair those tears. With adequate protein and adequate energy, the body rebuilds them. Your muscle grows bigger, so the next time you're working out, you'll have to increase the weight to tear the muscles again. If you did 10 kilos at the bench press last week, this week do 11 kilos. That tears your chest muscles a tiny bit more, and then your body responds by relaying more muscle. Next week, do 12 kilos, and it will tear a little bit more, and so on.

If you kept it at 10 kilos, your chest muscles would say, "I don't need to get any bigger now because all you're asking me to do is 10 kilos. I can do that." The muscle doesn't keep progressing, whereas if you asked it to do more, it would say, "If you want to lift 12 kilos now, we better get bigger." The muscles then get bigger and stronger so you can take it to the next level. The muscles now say, "If you want to lift 15 kilos, I better get bigger." This is called progressive overload training, and it's the basis of what all weight-lifting programs are based on.

By working your muscle to fatigue, you stimulate the muscular adaptation that will improve the metabolic capability of the muscle and cause it to grow. I recommend using four or five basic compound movements for your exercise set since compound movements target multiple muscle groups. These exercises can be enhanced for more difficulty by adding weights. I recommend the following five movements: squats, bench press, shoulder press, dead lifts, and pull-ups or chin-ups.

I remember a story about progressive overload training from university that has stuck with me ever since. Nearly 2,500 years ago, there was a man of incredible strength and athleticism roaming the hills of southern Italy. His name was Milo of Croton, and he was the most successful wrestler of his day. It is said that Milo built his incredible strength through a simple but profound strategy. One day, a newborn calf was born near his home. The wrestler decided to lift the small animal up and carry it on his shoulders. The next day, he returned and did the same. Milo continued this strategy for the next four years, hoisting the calf onto his shoulders each day as it grew, until he was no longer lifting a calf, but a four-year-old bull.

Every day, he would carry a heavier and heavier calf and noticed his legs, arms, and back were growing bigger. He realised that lifting something heavier every day would make his muscles grow. Most weight lifters follow some variation of this. There's a huge business in marketing the best way to build muscle, but it all ends up being the same. Just find something that you like and that works for you. What's important is to start, even if you're a complete beginner.

Let's go back to our friend, Susie, again. She scours the Internet for a month, trying to find the perfect way to put on muscle, whereas Jane, her best mate, skips the researching and simply starts doing movements she hasn't done before. Jane doesn't have the patience to research online and says, "To hell with that. I'm going to go to the gym for the next month." Jane's doing something that's making a difference. She might not follow a specific program, but she's experimenting—maybe doing some push-ups and then some lunges. She's going to see improvement because she's doing something she's never done before, moving her body in new ways. Those lunges soon become effortless, so Jane decides to step it up a notch and carry some weights in her hands, still doing the same amount of lunges. The added weights make them more challenging, and her quads are slowly growing stronger due to the increased stress. Jane is progressing as she experiments and tries to do more each week, whereas Susie's still at home scouring the Internet for the perfect program. Once Susie finally lands on a program she likes, she's now a month behind Jane, who simply started moving and challenging her body. I find it hilarious when people won't go to the gym until they've found the perfect program; they're wasting their time—any program they find is a variation of progressive overload. If you're that person who has consistently put off lifting weights, go and do it. Lifting weights doesn't have to be complicated. Just do a series of lower-body exercises, which use almost every muscle group from your hip down, followed by a series of upper-body exercises, which use almost every muscle group in the upper body. You certainly don't need a gym membership to get started. Squats don't have to be done underneath a squat rack. Start sitting down to a chair and standing up—it can be as simple as that. You don't need special equipment. Instead of the bench press, do push-ups.

A strength-training program doesn't change much between males or females. I'll caveat that by saying most females do predominantly want a better-looking bum and smaller thighs, so they can perform exercises that focus on those areas, but at the end of the day, the same principles apply. Just because Bob is trying to build muscle and Susie is trying to lose weight doesn't mean those programs need to be vastly different. I'd still include bench presses, chin-ups, squats, and dead lifts for both. There could be micro changes in these programs, depending on an individual's specific goals, but at the end of the day, if you want to put lean muscle mass on, you need to lift heavy things.

WHY WE STILL NEED CARDIO

Although cardiovascular activities on their own are pretty ineffective for pure weight loss, they are beneficial because they elevate your heart rate while working large muscles in your body. Participating in regular cardiovascular exercise has a plethora of other benefits for overall health. It reduces your risk for diabetes, lowers bad cholesterol, raises good cholesterol, increases feel-good chemicals in your brain, improves your circulation, and lowers your heart rate. It also helps in preventing heart attacks and strokes and fights against type 2 diabetes. Your heart is a muscle, and as such, it also gets a workout when you participate in cardiovascular exercise. As you jog around the block, your heart pumps blood through your body at a more rapid pace, which in turn increases the flow by about four times from its resting rate. Your breathing also increases, and your muscles get a higher dose of oxygen. You don't see a hell of a lot of marathon runners dying of cardiovascular disease, type 2 diabetes, or strokes. Overall, if you look at the population, I guarantee you there's far less of a percentage of marathon runners dying of heart attacks than average people.

There are so many other intrinsic benefits you can't see when you consistently engage in cardiovascular movement. When you walk up a hill, for example, you won't feel as winded or tired because your cardiovascular system is much better. Cardio should be included in your life, and it can be as simple as walking. Some people think cardio means intense activities, like running for ten kilometers or biking for one hundred kilometers, and that the intensity needs to be on the verge of vomiting. It doesn't. I think people get these ideas from shows like *The Biggest Loser*. A simple forty-minute walk can have huge benefits for your cardiovascular system.

Whether you walk a kilometer or run a kilometer, it uses the exact same amount of energy. It all boils down to physics: mass over distance. Running takes a lot less time compared to walking. If you walked ten kilometers, it might take you half a day, whereas if you ran the same distance, it would take you an hour and a half. If time isn't a factor, you don't have to run. I have clients who ask me all the time, "Don't I have to run?" If time is not a factor for you and you hate running, go for a walk, but make sure to go the same distance as you would if you ran so that you use the same energy. Most of us complain that time is against us, and we don't have enough of it, which is why I suggest running as a beneficial activity to do.

It's about finding something you enjoy. If you're not a runner, don't run. I personally think running is the greatest gift we were ever given. It's a complete equaliser in that I've seen African men who had no shoes run a marathon at the Olympics. You don't need to have the best sports institutes or the best scientists to figure out the best running techniques in order to advance to the Olympics, because the sport is simple: Put on a pair of shoes, and run. I love running; it's economical, it's easy to do, and you don't need special equipment or a gym. You can simply open your front door and go. Cycling, in contrast, has other costs associated with it. The bike, helmet, bike shorts, and shoes costs money. You also have to find bike paths because a lot of people don't like riding on the road with cars. There are all sorts of hindrances to other sports compared to running. If you like swimming, you'll certainly need a body of water. Whatever it might be, find a cardio exercise that you enjoy doing. The diet that works best is the one that you stick to; it's the same with cardiovascular training. Find the thing that works best for you. If you don't know what you like, experiment and find it. There's running, biking, swimming, rowing, walking, climbing, hiking—anything you can think of that raises your heart rate. It doesn't have to be anything intense where you find yourself ill at the end of the session. You don't have to lie in a puddle of sweat at the end of thirty minutes. I want people to get away from the CrossFit mentality of going balls out, that it's all or nothing. You don't have to do that in order to get a good workout in. Focus on moving your body in a way that you don't normally move it, and do that for a period of at least a half hour to an hour. If spewing in a corner doing CrossFit is enjoyable to you, awesome. Go sign up at your local CrossFit and do it. I don't begrudge CrossFit at all; I think it's a fantastic option for taking your fitness to the next level—if that's what you're into. For Susie who's starting out, that can be terrifying, so I would never send Susie to CrossFit, because she'd do it once, throw up, and not be able to walk for three days. She'd never exercise again. She'll think, *If that's what it takes for me to lose weight, nuh-uh. That's not for me.*

It's important to note that if you're a beginner, be sure to start small. Ease into your cardio and strength training.

Don't say, "I'm going to start running today," and instead of doing a two-minute run around the block as a starting point, you go run five kilometers. You won't be able to walk comfortably for five days after, and so you'll say something defeatist like, "See? Running's not for me. I can't even move my legs. That's just stupid. I'm never going to run again." Start small. Run around the block. Tomorrow, do two laps. Next week, do four laps. Start small, and progress as you improve over time.

"How much should I be exercising?" is a common question I hear. I suggest engaging in movement four days out of each week, but it depends on the person and his or her goals. For people who have never exercised before, two to three strength training sessions a week and a walk or two is more than enough.

People always say to me, "You must be training seven days a week to maintain the body you're sporting." I love their facial expressions when I tell them I only train three days a week. It's true—that's all I do. Now, mind you, it's taken me a long time to get to that point. My current goals are to maintain, so training three days a week is sufficient enough because I'm not trying to get bigger or lose weight (although I could always do with bigger biceps). If I wanted to take my body to the next level, like a bodybuilder for example, I'd be in the gym a little bit more than I currently am.

DON'T FORGET TO REST

Resting days are an integral part of the process. The changes in your body need time to repair themselves, and they can't do that without a break. Because lifting weights or doing body-weight exercises such as squats, lunges, or push-ups microtear your muscles, your body needs time to recover. According to the American College of Sports Medicine, a rest day must occur at least one to two times per week. These rest days are a key part of any exercise program, and they're vital for positive results and a reduction in injury risk. If you want to go for a walk with your spouse or dog, you certainly can, but you don't have to. Feel free to sit on the couch and enjoy a rest day as long as, throughout the week, you've put in the work.

7

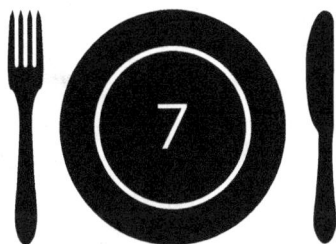

HAPPINESS IS THE END GAME

Having the body of your dreams will never bring you happiness. You might think it will, but it's not fulfilling enough. Taking care of yourself will increase your happiness—you certainly have to take care of yourself when working toward a ripped body—but happiness is in your mind, not in your muscles.

I experienced a powerfully humbling moment when I signed a new client once. He came in, and I asked him the same series of questions I ask all my clients, one of which was, "Who's your celebrity crush?" I do this not because I think my program will necessarily help them look like said crush, but it is good for me to know where

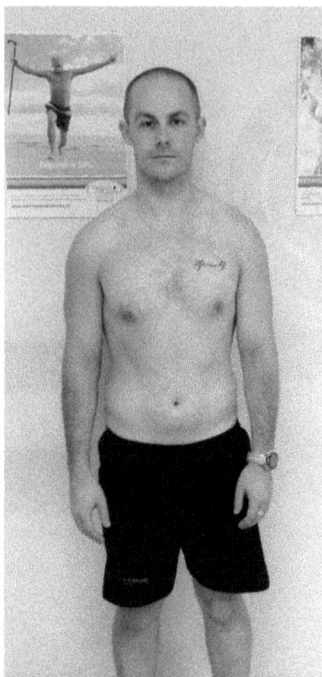

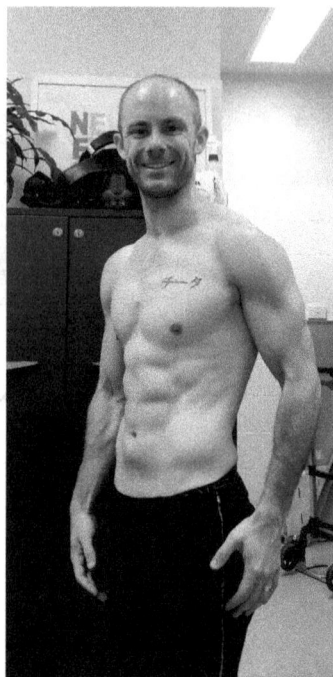

the client's head is and what he or she finds appealing and attractive; this then allows me to build a program that is specific to his or her needs. His answer: "Well, if I'm to be honest, mate, I've been following you on Snapchat, and the picture of yourself that you posted last week—well, I want to look like that."

I did my best to compose myself and not react like a giddy little girl with an "Oh, my god! Oh, my god! Oh, my god! He thinks I have a great body!" kind of thing.

Because I'm professional, I held it together and said, "That's so flattering. Thank you."

But truly, on the inside, I went, "Oh, my god! Oh, my god! Oh, my god!"

Here I had a client telling me, "I want to look like you," but when I woke up that morning and looked in the mirror, I said to myself, "I don't look like Zac Efron on the set of *Bay Watch*." Having a body people aspire to is flattering, and even though the body I've worked for is something I am incredibly proud of, it certainly isn't the beholder of my happiness. Chasing your dream body or losing weight won't make you happy, and it's the wrong way to look at things. To repeat what we covered in chapter 1, happiness is the thing that you need to find first. Once you discover what that is, everything else—and this includes sculpting your dream body—falls in behind that.

Happiness for Bob might be spending more time with his kids and not working so much and going on a holiday every couple of months. These things make him happy because he values his family and time off, and they don't cause any stress. A content mind-set puts him in a much better place to engage in a weight-loss program and then chase those dreams of feeling and looking better.

Happiness leads to weight loss. Weight loss does not necessarily lead to happiness.

Ever heard of Gary Vaynerchuk? He's a successful entrepreneur whom Mike Vacanti used to train. Gary works eighteen hours a day, and he loves it. To me, that sounds like hell. If I worked eighteen hours a day, I would be a miserable person, but for him, that's his game; that's what he loves. He's the type of guy who finds sleeping annoying because it takes time away from working.

I'm guessing you're like me, however, and you're looking for more balance in your life. Whatever happiness is for you, find that first.

We live in a world these days that is predicated on social media telling us that unless you're a millionaire, unless you have the body of Zac Efron, unless you have five cars and a big house, you are a failure. We have to recalibrate what we consider a failure because that's absurd.

Gary Vaynerchuk talks about this, too. He gave an example using the top 1 percent of earners in America. The minimum salary to be considered a part of that top 1 percent is $400,000 a year, yet when you survey people and ask them how much they think those people earn, their answer is an absurd $10,000,000 or more a year. That's a perception we're creating. You might be sitting at home trying to start your business, aspiring to be the top 1 percent in the world, all the while thinking you have to make $1,000,000 when the reality is a lot less than that. Don't stress yourself out thinking, "I'm a failure because I only make $350,000 a year." No, you're above 98 percent of the population. That's like being Usain Bolt at the Olympics.

What makes you happy? If you hate your job and you hate your life, I give you full respect if you stay with it because you have a mortgage and other bills to pay, but I'm sorry, the reality is you're wasting your time if you think you don't have another choice. I would leave that job in an instant. I would find a way to leave it. If you can't quit your job right now, that's fine, but there are many other hours outside of your job that you could be spending on something that would put you in the right place in six months' time. Maybe you can quit your job in eighteen months and start living that life you've always dreamt of.

My passion is helping people live happier, healthier, and longer lives. My sister inspired me to write this book, and now I want to see it get into as many hands as possible because, deep down in my core, I believe it can make a difference and help a million people—who knows, maybe even ten million!

HAPPINESS IS NOT ON SOCIAL MEDIA

We also mistakenly take our cues for happiness and what it looks like from social media. Social media is usually a highlight reel of people's lives, and most people don't post the struggles they're going through. We're generally too plugged in, which makes our stress levels skyrocket as we constantly compare our lives to the lives of others, thinking theirs are better. The grass on the other side is often not as green as we tend to think it is.

I think social media is hugely positive for the most part, but it plays into that "unless you are this, you are a failure" mentality. There's an invisible and unrealistic bar that has been set because many people see posts from others and automatically assume they are successful, whether that's because they posted a photo of a fancy car, a big house, or wads of cash. I don't believe most of those posts are even remotely close to the truth. I bet people go to the bank to pull out $50,000 of the only money they have, lay it over the bed, and take a selfie, or they take a photo in a Ferrari they hired out, saying, "I have the secrets to business success. Follow me, and I'll get you there." This idea of "I'm successful because I own a Ferrari and have $50,000 laying on my bed" is simply ridiculous. We're being brainwashed into thinking others are happy, and since you might not have this, that, or the other as they do, then your life is worthless. It's hard to get out of that negative headspace when that message is constantly flooding our social-media streams.

You have to recalibrate what happiness is for you. If it is owning a Ferrari, fine. Go and do something to make that dream a reality. Don't sit there and complain that you don't have a Ferrari.

Instead of going out to eat every Friday, my wife and I save up, and once every three months, we splurge on ourselves and eat a fancy meal together. I think we're probably still ahead in cost when you compare it to those who go out every single Friday, but lots of people are quick to judge and make assumptions saying, "You must be so wealthy if you're spending $500 a head on dinner." No, the reality is that we haven't done anything but sit at home and eat chicken and vegetables (and ice cream) every night, so we can afford that.

Don't let these types of things distract you from the little things in life. I enjoy social media, and I'm an active participant because it's fun and it's a way for me to reach more people, but I don't let it consume me or distract me from what is important in my life. For example, I completely unplug when I'm at home and I'm with my daughter and wife. I've never found love like I've found with my daughter, and I want to cherish every moment

I have as she grows up. I could have the worst day of my life at the office, but the moment I get home and I see her smiling, it's not a bad day anymore. Everything that made my day miserable immediately becomes trivial. For me, I'm all about family, and when I get to spend time with them, I'm happy. Put your happiness above social media, and stop judging yourself based on the highlight reels of other people.

HAPPINESS COMES FROM WITHIN

If you want to find your happy place, you need to create it. You can sit there and wallow in your own pity that the world is against you and everything's difficult, but to quote Gary Vaynerchuk again, "If anyone who looks like you has done it before, then you can, too." The alternative is you can continue to sit there and complain for the rest of your life and be miserable.

With full respect, I understand that people have various challenges that pop up in their lives, but what's the alternative? To sit stagnant and complain? I disagree with that kind of mentality and find it counterintuitive. I've worked with plenty of clients who have often complained about their lives or offered excuses about why they didn't do something I asked them to. "Oh, I worked late last night, and I wasn't able to do the foam-rolling you told me to do."

"My newborn was crying, and I was up all night feeding her, so I couldn't plan my meals like I should have."

"My boyfriend broke up with me."

"My boss needed a report first thing the next morning, and I didn't have time to get to the gym."

"I was running late, so I grabbed McDonald's on the way to work."

"I was tired."

Blah, blah, blah. Come on! It really gets up my nerve. After more than ten years running my business and hearing every excuse under the sun, they all fall on deaf ears. I have a lot less patience for that kind of talk these days than I used to. I fully respect that your life is difficult, but it could be worse. Things could always be worse.

PRACTICING MINDFULNESS

I can be a fairly stressed-out individual at times. Most of us are more stressed out than we are not. Practicing mindful activities can help ground ourselves, which then helps us find happiness, which then helps us in our fitness goals.

I think meditation is key to finding balance. And I don't mean the stereotypical meditation often depicted on television where you sit for an hour, humming away (at least that's the mental picture I get when I think about meditation). It can be as simple as putting your phone away, closing the computer, turning the TV off, and closing your eyes for ten minutes.

I enjoy meditating, and it's amazing how much clearer and how much more destressed my thoughts become when I shut the world off for five or ten minutes. I've come across a heap of apps that talk you through a meditation, bringing you down and relaxing your brain. I used to be a skeptic, too. I was that guy who laughed at people when they said, "Calm your thoughts, and think of a distant beach somewhere." Blah. "Whatever!" I would say. "I don't need that crap to wind me down. I know how to wind down." But they do genuinely work, and it's a powerful skill to develop.

You don't have to practise standard meditation, either. I think meditation can be found in a variety of activities, and it goes back to what you like and what works for you. Yoga is a great form of meditation. Yoga focuses on your breathing and movement of the body in a way that is calming and strengthening. I've seen big, bulky guys who start doing yoga, and they see vast improvements in the gym; they're more supple and more clear with their thoughts. There are some strong dudes who only practise yoga as their strength training. Others find meditation in running, cycling, or swimming. Even lifting weights can be a form of meditation, as long as you focus and don't let outside influences distract you. Whatever it might be for you, meditation is where you can calm your thoughts and hone in on that mind-and-body connection.

What things are mindful for you? The moment I get home, I switch it all off because I want to be present with my wife and daughter. Seeing my two girls recharges me. I also find running mindful. When I run, I don't take my phone with me, and I don't listen to music. Find what's mindful for you, and practise it as often as you can. Whatever it might be, you need to find what disconnects you from this stressful and manic world. It could be two to three times a day if you can prioritise time for it, but unplug as often as you can, and switch off and get out of your work space, your head space, and your social-media space.

CATCH THOSE ZS

Sleep is the most underrated part of any weight-loss program. Without quality sleep, there's no way you can operate at your full potential. The average person should sleep between seven and eight hours—some can manage with less, while some need more—but it's also the quality of sleep that needs to be taken into consideration. You can assess your sleeping patterns with smartphone applications that track your sleep to find out if you're getting the sleep your body and mind needs.

What's interesting from the science perspective is that scientists have yet to concretely discover and explain why we sleep. There's no physiological reason why we need to sleep, since we provide our bodies energy with the food we eat, so it's not an energy thing. Some believe we need to sleep because it functions as a reset button—sort of like when your computer is on day after day and it gets a bit chuggy. Once you reset it, it tends to run a bit better. It's the same for us in that if we're awake and moving around all day, we get a bit run down and need a break.

When we sleep, some scientists believe our system shuts down so our brain can focus on filing away all the things we did that day. It's as if our brains are saying, "We've learned ten different things over the last ten days, so let's put that bit into long-term memory, let's pull this memory and put it there..." What do computers do? They defrag and put things away in folders in different places. Some scientists believe that's what we do when we sleep, but there's no concrete evidence to back that up; it's only a theory. All we know is that sleeping is crucial to our well-being, our psychology, and our physiology. If you're not getting enough of it, you need to address it.

YOUR FITNESS JOURNEY NEVER ENDS

Later-day eating changed my sister's life, not only physically but emotionally and circumstantially as well—and the journey isn't over. It's a never-ending process of putting the work in, day in and day out, for the rest of your life.

I shared the story of my sister achieving her goal weight before her holiday to Europe. When she arrived at the airport, she weighed twenty-seven kilos lighter since starting the Start Late, Stay Light lifestyle. The limit for luggage when traveling overseas is twenty-three kilos. When the check-in staff asked her to lift her bag onto the scales, she could barely do it; her bag weighed eighteen kilos.

A big light bulb went off in her head, and she called me in tears.

"I didn't realise how much my body was suffering over the last decade or so. My bag for Europe weighed eighteen kilos, which I could barely lift myself, and my body had to carry that weight, plus another eight on top of that, for more than ten years. No wonder I felt like shit."

Before starting the program, Sarah accepted her reality of losing her breath a little standing up from the couch or climbing some stairs. She thought it was normal: *Well, this is how it is.* No. Just because you might be used to the way your body reacts to something, that doesn't mean that it's a normal reaction. People underestimate how much kilos actually weigh. Someone says, "Oh, I've only lost five kilos," as if it's not a big deal. Let me give you a five-kilo plate and tell you to hold it for the next twenty-four hours; you'll quickly realise how hard it is to carry that extra weight around. Unnecessary extra weight is incredibly taxing on your body, but people become used to it because the weight is put on gradually.

That airport experience helped put my sister's journey into perspective. She realised how much those extra kilos impacted her body. If only I could put that little epiphany in a bottle and share it with others, I think everyone would succeed. When someone is having a tough time six weeks in, and they've only lost three kilos, I wish I could open that bottle and say, "Drink this. Know what it will feel like to be stronger, healthier, and lighter." Here's a brief reflection from my sister:

> *Start Late, Stay Light has given my life back (and may have even saved my life). In the beginning, I had a lot of doubt and some real rough weeks dealing with the scales*

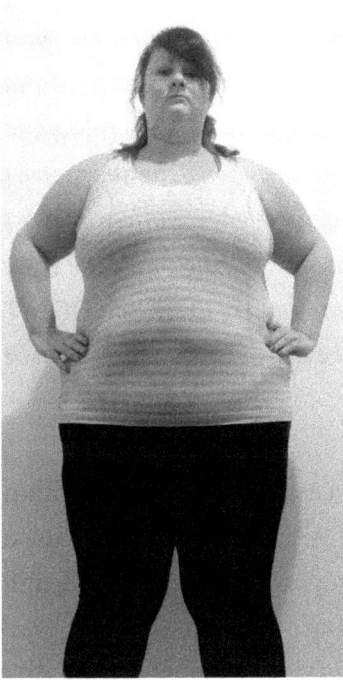

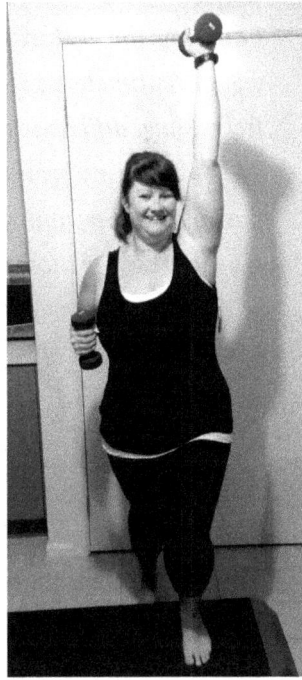

not moving (despite sticking to the program to the T) as well as dealing with my own inner monologue telling me to just stop and give up. I'm sure you've all had that little voice telling you to just stop.

But now that little voice has changed its tune and is telling me to keep going. It tells me how proud it is of me. I can't say I find this "easy," but as the weeks tick over, I do find it easier to keep going. When I first started, I had a goal weight I wanted to get to before my first overseas trip to Europe, and I did it!

I am now down thirty-two kilograms and more than eighty centimeters in just thirty-seven weeks! I see and feel the huge difference it has made to me and my life, and I can't thank my brother, Adam, enough for the support, pushing, and encouragement he gave me over the past six months. For those who are hearing that little voice telling you to give up, then I'm here to tell you DON'T LISTEN! It won't always be easy, but I promise it will be worth it in the end!

My sister has seen great success on this program within the first thirty-seven weeks, and as she continues to lose weight, she will continue to improve her life and her health on this endless fitness journey.

You, too, can create a better life for yourself. Work on being a better version of yourself, and know that you're strong, powerful, and capable. You can do this!

I have said it before, and I will continue to say it: If you don't have health, you don't have much. What if you were told that today was the last day of your life? Would you worry about not buying a Lamborghini (I might be, but that's just me) or living in a big house? If I were told that tomorrow was my last day on earth because a bus would hit and kill me, I'd go straight home to spend every last minute with my family.

What if you could live another twenty years into your senior years healthy, capable, and strong? That means twenty more years to spend with kids and grandkids, twenty more years to travel the world, twenty more years to work on your dreams. On your deathbed at age ninety, looking back at your life, I'd be willing to bet you'd be happy because you did the things you wanted to do and watched your kids and grandkids grow up. All people on their deathbed always say they wished they'd spent more time with their families. "I wish" is the number-one thing they always start with, whether it's "I wish I spent more time with my family" or "I wish I went on that holiday." It's never "I wish I built a $1,000,000,000 company," or "I wish I had a Lamborghini," or "I wish I had worked more."

If you have health, you're going to have more time to live your dreams, whatever they might be. If I can give Susie twenty extra years of her life to pursue those dreams, I think that's worth fighting for, as opposed to her going about her life and dying at age fifty-five from a heart attack.

This lifestyle is your key to that happier, healthier, and longer life. Start Late, Stay Light is a tried-and-true way to help you achieve whatever goals you're looking to achieve—whether that's weight loss, improved health, feeling better, or leading a happier, more engaged life with no regrets on your deathbed. This lifestyle is just that—a lifestyle. You have to commit to it for the long haul in order to fully reap the benefits. Naturally, you will have good days and bad days—we are all human—but don't you dare quit when things get hard. You deserve to give yourself the best gift in life: good health. Keep going when you don't want to, get back on track when you fall off, trust yourself, and trust the process.

I'll be right here rooting for you every step of the way.

SIXTEEN-WEEK PROGRAMS

TESTIMONIALS FROM WOMEN

ASH, 28

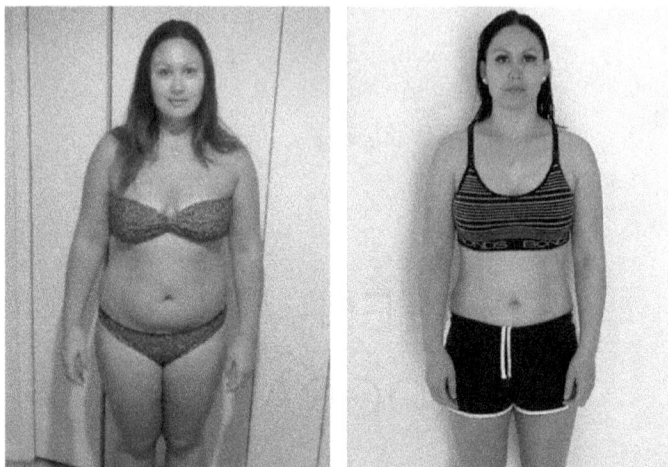

Adam, thank you for going above and beyond in providing support for me on my weight-loss journey. You have not only pushed me to reach my goals but have taught me that this lifestyle is sustainable and achievable. Knowing I have daily support from others on the program has made me want to aim high, even though the only person I'm competing with is myself. Your program has given me the drive I've needed to finally achieve my goal of more than eight years—and for that, I will be forever grateful. Jo-Lo body, here I come!

RHIAN, 38

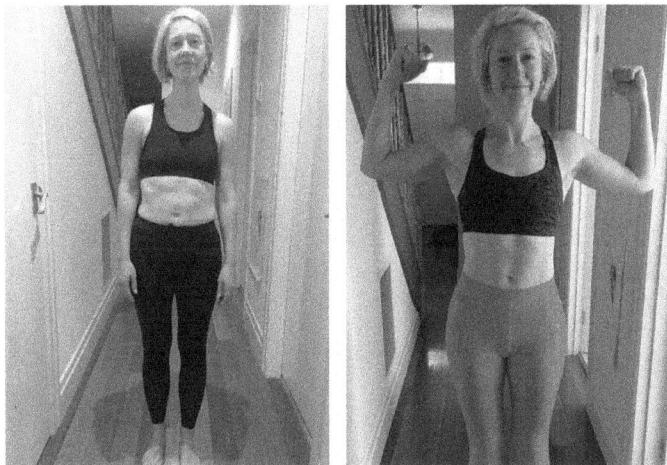

The Start Late, Stay Light program gave me an excellent framework to regain control of what and how much I was eating. I was surprised at how easily I transitioned to the later-day eating lifestyle. I won't lie: The first day or two took a bit of getting used to, but after that, it was easy. My diet wasn't terrible before, but I needed to lose a few kilos, and this program helped me do that. I began losing body fat in the first week without giving up all the sweet treats I love. Tracking what I ate every day taught me to be more mindful of my eating habits without being obsessive. The Start Late, Stay Light program is a lifestyle change and not a diet, so I don't feel like I am missing out on the good things in life. More importantly, it is a sustainable way of living. I'm not quite where I want to be yet, but thanks to the Start Late, Stay Light program, I am well on my way! Best of all, there are no "cheat" days, which means I never feel guilty. It's perfect!

BERNADETTE, 47

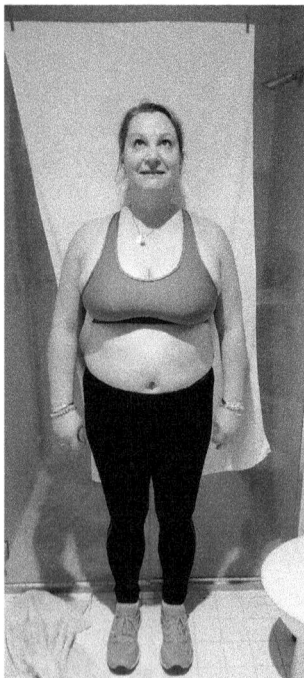

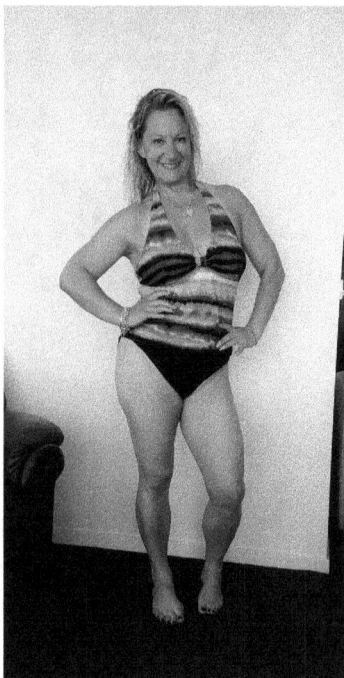

I was a strong believer that the best way to start your day was with a healthy and low GI breakfast. When I spoke to Adam during our initial phone call and he told me that my first meal wouldn't be until 1:00 p.m., I must admit I panicked! I thought to myself, "What is this guy thinking? Breakfast is the most important meal of the day! How is this going to work?" I admit the first few days were difficult, but my body quickly adjusted, and the results started soon after. I began this journey on 9 October 2016, and to date I've lost close to sixteen kilos. I feel incredible, and everybody tells me that I look great. The Start Late, Stay Light eating plan works wonders, so be brave and take the journey—you won't regret it! Thank you, Adam!

SIXTEEN-WEEK PROGRAM FOR AVERAGE SUSIE

Meet Susie. She's your average woman. Perhaps you're like Susie and you sit in an office for work or you're a stay-at-home mum with a few kids to look after. Perhaps you've been looking to lose a little weight and want to find a way to cook healthy foods, not only for yourself, but also for your family, so you don't have to cook separate meals for everyone. If your numbers fall within Average Susie's range, follow the exercise and food plan in the subsequent pages. If you are outside of these ranges, email me, and I will happily give you some suggestions on how you could change this food plan to work for you. These numbers reflect an average height, weight, and body fat percentage for this segment of the population.

Age: 20 to 60
Height: 150 cm to 170 cm
Weight: 65 kg to 80kg
Body Fat Percentage: 30-50%
Calories: 1200 kcal to 1400 kcal
Protein: 115 g to 135 g
Carbohydrates: 120 g to 125 g
Fats: 30 g to 40 g

Make sure you track your weight and measurements each week to see how your body reacts to the meal plan and the amount of food you are eating. Measure your chest, waist, and hips each week, and write the numbers down. If you're losing a lot of weight and feeling hungry, you might want to add a little more food into your plan. If you're not seeing any results after a few weeks and you followed the program to the letter, then look to reduce the amount of food until you begin to see some results come through.

You may start strength training right from the start in order to build the habit, if you'd like, but it is not 100 percent necessary in the first four weeks. You should, however, engage in some cardiovascular activities. This could be walking during your lunch break, parking further away from your office and walking, or hand-delivering a message to a work colleague across the office instead of sending an email. We'll start heavily incorporating strength training when we reach week five. You'll be lifting two to three times per week and supplementing the other two to three days with activities such as walking, swimming, yoga, Pilates, or cycling.

From weeks nine to twelve, strength training should be an integral part of your weekly routine with two to three sessions combined with one high-intensity interval training (HIIT) session a week. Your usual light cardiovascular activities such as walking, swimming, yoga, Pilates, or cycling should continue to fill in on the days you're not strength training.

Reaching the last phase from weeks thirteen to sixteen, you should have developed a solid routine of exercise, great food, fun, and fitness. By the end of this stage, you should have dropped some weight and centimeters, but more importantly, you should be feeling better about yourself.

Once you complete this stage, congratulations! You are now an official later-day eater and are well on your way to living a happy, healthy, and longer life. Welcome to the later-day eating tribe! The journey isn't over, though. Take what you've learned, and begin to work those skills into the next twenty, thirty, forty, or fifty years of your life. This is a lifelong pursuit and one that will always have its ups and downs, challenging you at every turn. With the skills developed through this program, however, you have the confidence to tackle any obstacle head-on, continuing to see results forever.

Later-day eaters for *life*!

AVERAGE SUSIE WEEKS ONE TO FOUR: PREPARATION PHASE

The focus during this phase is to develop a routine of not eating in the morning, pushing your first meal until you have achieved a sixteen-hour fasting window and a six- to eight-hour feasting window. I'm not too concerned about what you eat in this stage, since the main focus should be on pushing your first meal to about 1:00 in the afternoon. Although not mandatory (yet), I highly recommend downloading a macro-tracking application on your phone (like MyFitnessPal) and starting to track what you eat in order to familiarise yourself with and learn more about the foods you love.

AVERAGE SUSIE WEEKS ONE TO FOUR: TRAINING PROGRAMS

As you know, strength training is crucial to your overall success on this program. You must include these workouts into your weekly routine, as they will not only help with weight loss, but they will also help to increase your lean muscle mass, which will in turn keep you strong and mobile throughout your journey.

The training program for the first four weeks can be done at home or at a gym and only require a couple of dumbbells (DB) for some of the upper-body exercises. Make sure you track your workouts to ensure you are seeing week-to-week progress and pushing yourself to improve.

With each program, aim to complete the exercises as one big circuit, performing each exercise in the set with no rests. Rest for 90 seconds in between each set.

Follow this program for the first four weeks, but feel free to swap days in order to work with your schedule. Make sure you have adequate time to recover; rest days are as important as training days.

Monday: Program 1
Tuesday: Long Walk or Run (more than 30 minutes)
Wednesday: Rest Day (could do a yoga or Pilates class)
Thursday: Program 2
Friday: Complete Rest Day
Saturday: Program 3
Sunday: Long Walk or Run (more than 30 minutes)

AVERAGE SUSIE WEEKS ONE TO FOUR: PROGRAM 1

EXERCISE	SETS	REPS	WEIGHT
Squats	1	10 to 15	N/A to Light
	2	10 to 15	N/A to Light
	3	10 to 15	N/A to Light
Stationary Lunge	1	10 to 15	N/A to Light
	2	10 to 15	N/A to Light
	3	10 to 15	N/A to Light
Sumo DB Squat	1	10 to 15	N/A to Light
	2	10 to 15	N/A to Light
	3	10 to 15	N/A to Light
Glute Bridge Raise	1	10 to 15	N/A
	2	10 to 15	N/A
	3	10 to 15	N/A
Step-Ups	1	10 to 15	N/A to Light
	2	10 to 15	N/A to Light
	3	10 to 15	N/A to Light
Wall Squat Hold	1	30 s to 60 s	N/A
	2	30 s to 60 s	N/A
	3	30 s to 60 s	N/A
Rest (90 s)			

AVERAGE SUSIE WEEKS ONE TO FOUR: PROGRAM 2

EXERCISE	SETS	REPS	WEIGHT
Push-Ups	1	10 to 15	N/A
	2	10 to 15	N/A
	3	10 to 15	N/A
Seated Shoulder Press	1	10 to 15	Light
	2	10 to 15	Light
	3	10 to 15	Light
Dips	1	10 to 15	N/A
	2	10 to 15	N/A
	3	10 to 15	N/A
Seated Bicep Curl	1	10 to 15	Light
	2	10 to 15	Light
	3	10 to 15	Light
Lying DB Pullover	1	10 to 15	Light
	2	10 to 15	Light
	3	10 to 15	Light
DB 1 Arm Row	1	10 to 15	Light
	2	10 to 15	Light
	3	10 to 15	Light
Rest (90 s)			

AVERAGE SUSIE WEEKS ONE TO FOUR: PROGRAM 3

EXERCISE	SETS	REPS	WEIGHT
Dual Knee Tuck	1	10 to 15	N/A
	2	10 to 15	N/A
	3	10 to 15	N/A
Alternating V-Snap	1	10 to 15	N/A
	2	10 to 15	N/A
	3	10 to 15	N/A
Cycle Legs	1	10 to 15	N/A
	2	10 to 15	N/A
	3	10 to 15	N/A
Toe Touches	1	10 to 15	N/A
	2	10 to 15	N/A
	3	10 to 15	N/A
Russian Twist	1	10 to 15	N/A
	2	10 to 15	N/A
	3	10 to 15	N/A
Plank Hold	1	30 s to 60 s	N/A
	2	30 s to 60 s	N/A
	3	30 s to 60 s	N/A
Rest (90 s)			

AVERAGE SUSIE WEEKS FIVE TO EIGHT: MOMENTUM PHASE

This is the phase where most people fall off the wagon, so pay close attention to your emotional state and to how your body is feeling, and steer away from stressful situations. Stay the course, and should you have a day where it doesn't go to plan, always remember that you are only one meal or workout away from getting back on track. Don't let one bad meal or one missed workout turn into an entire weekend or week of missed meals and workouts.

AVERAGE SUSIE WEEKS FIVE TO EIGHT MEAL PLAN

Use the following meal plans for the first four weeks. Feel free to change the days around, should it be easier to prepare the meals in a different order.

MONDAY

Calories: 1200 kcal to 1400 kcal
Protein: 115 g to 135g
Carbs: 120 g to 125 g
Fats: 30 g to 40 g

MEAL ONE

Salad Items of Choice: Spinach, Tomato, Grated Carrot, Sliced Beetroot, Cucumber, Spanish Onion
3 x Small Tins of Tuna in Spring Water
     or
180 g Skin-Off Chicken Breast (oven baked)
     or
180 g Lean-Beef Stir-Fry Strips (minimal oil used to cook)
Salt, Pepper, and Fresh Lemon Juice for Seasoning
Salt, Pepper, and Fresh Lemon Juice for Seasoning

MEAL TWO

1 x Banana

1 x Pink Lady Apple

MEAL THREE

Pizza:

1 x Wholemeal Lite Lebanese/Pita Bread as Base

50 g Tomato Paste

150 g Shaved Lean Leg Ham

50 g Pineapple

50 g Mushrooms

50 g Light Tasty Shredded Cheese

Drink plenty of water.

TUESDAY

Calories: 1200 kcal to 1400 kcal

Protein: 115 g to 135 g

Carbs: 120 g to 125 g

Fats: 30 g to 40 g

MEAL ONE

Salad Items of Choice: Spinach, Tomato, Grated Carrot, Sliced Beetroot, Cucumber, Spanish Onion

3 x Small Tins of Tuna in Spring Water
  or
180 g Skin-Off Chicken Breast (oven baked)
  or
180 g Lean-Beef Stir-Fry Strips (minimal oil used to cook)
Salt, Pepper, Seasoning

MEAL TWO

Protein Shake (make sure your protein powder is 75%–80% protein with nominal carbohydrates and fats):
30 g Scoop of Favourite-Flavour Protein Powder Mixed with Water
1 x Orange

MEAL THREE

2 Lean Beef Mince Burgers (add favourite herbs and seasonings)
2 Lite Wholemeal, Soft Wraps
20 ml Heinz Ketchup per Wrap
Salad Items of Choice: Spinach, Tomato, Grated Carrot, Sliced Beetroot, Cucumber, Spanish Onion (no cheese)
Drink plenty of water.

WEDNESDAY

Calories: 1200 kcal to 1400 kcal
Protein: 115 g to 135 g
Carbs: 120 g to 125 g
Fats: 30 g to 40 g

MEAL ONE

Salad Items of Choice: Spinach, Tomato, Grated Carrot,
Sliced Beetroot, Cucumber, Spanish Onion
3 x Small Tins of Tuna in Spring Water
  or
180 g Skin-Off Chicken Breast (oven baked)
  or
180 g Lean-Beef Stir-Fry Strips (minimal oil used to
cook)
Salt, Pepper and Fresh Lemon Juice for Seasoning

MEAL TWO

Protein Shake (make sure your protein powder is 75%
–80% protein with nominal carbohydrates and fats):
30 g Scoop of Favourite-Flavour Protein Powder
1 x Banana
80 g Mixed Berries
Water, Ice Blended

MEAL THREE

Peri Peri Chicken and Roast Veggies
190 g Peri Peri Skin-Off Chicken Breast Steaks
100 g Sweet Potato
50 g Red Capsicum
30 g Carrots
0.5 tbsp Olive Oil (coat and roast veggies)
100 g Frozen Broccoli
Drink plenty of water.

THURSDAY

Calories: 1200 kcal to 1400 kcal
Protein: 115 g to 135 g
Carbs: 120 g to 125 g
Fats: 30 g to 40 g

MEAL ONE

Salad Items of Choice: Spinach, Tomato, Grated Carrot,
Sliced Beetroot, Cucumber, Spanish Onion
3 x Small Tins of Tuna in Spring Water
    or
180 g Skin-Off Chicken Breast (oven baked)
    or
180 g Lean-Beef Stir-Fry Strips (minimal oil used to cook)
Salt, Pepper, and Fresh Lemon Juice for Seasoning

MEAL TWO

1 x Orange

1 x Apple

1 x Cookies-and-Cream Quest Bar

MEAL THREE

200 g Porterhouse Steak (cut as much fat off as possible)

150 g Frozen Green Veggies

150 g Oven-Baked Straight Cut Chips

Drink plenty of water.

FRIDAY

Calories: 1200 kcal to 1400 kcal

Protein: 115 g to 135 g

Carbs: 120 g to 125 g

Fats: 30 g to 40 g

MEAL ONE

Salad Items of Choice: Spinach, Tomato, Grated Carrot, Sliced Beetroot, Cucumber, Spanish Onion

3 x Small Tins of Tuna in Spring Water

or

180 g Skin-Off Chicken Breast (oven baked)
or
180 g Lean-Beef Stir-Fry Strips (minimal oil used to cook)
Salt, Pepper, and Fresh Lemon Juice for Seasoning

MEAL TWO

1 x Orange
1 x Banana

MEAL THREE

Sunday Night Roast:
250 g Free-Range Chicken Rotisserie (remove all skin)
100 g Potato (roasted)
100 g Pumpkin (roasted)
1 tbsp of Olive Oil with Salt, Pepper, and Herbs
150 g Frozen Mixed Green Veggies
Drink plenty of water.

SATURDAY

Calories: 1200 kcal to 1400 kcal
Protein: 115 g to 135 g
Carbs: 120 g to 125 g
Fats: 30 g to 40 g

MEAL ONE

Salad Items of Choice: Spinach, Tomato, Grated Carrot, Sliced Beetroot, Cucumber, Spanish Onion

3 x Small Tins of Tuna in Spring Water

or

180 g Skin-Off Chicken Breast (oven baked)

or

180 g Lean-Beef Stir-Fry Strips (minimal oil used to cook)

Salt, Pepper, and Fresh Lemon Juice for Seasoning

MEAL TWO

1 x Banana

MEAL THREE

Jacket Potato and Taco Mince:

250 g 98% Lean-Beef Mince

350 g Passatta

1 Small Packet Taco Seasoning Mix

100 g Mushrooms

50 g Corn

250 g Potato (cook in microwave or oven, then pour mince mixture over the potato)

20 g Light Tasty Cheddar Cheese (sprinkle on potato)

Drink plenty of water.

SUNDAY

Calories: 1200 kcal to 1400 kcal
Protein: 115 g to 135 g
Carbs: 120 g to 125 g
Fats: 30 g to 40 g

MEAL ONE

Salad Items of Choice: Spinach, Tomato, Grated Carrot,
Sliced Beetroot, Cucumber, Spanish Onion
3 x Small Tins of Tuna in Spring Water
or
180 g Skin-Off Chicken Breast (oven baked)
or
180 g Lean-Beef Stir-Fry Strips (minimal oil used to
cook)
Salt, Pepper, and Fresh Lemon Juice for Seasoning

MEAL TWO

Protein Shake (make sure your protein powder is 75%–
80% protein with nominal carbohydrates and fats):
20 g Scoop of Favourite-Flavour Protein Powder
250 ml No-Fat Milk
200 g Punnet of Strawberries

MEAL THREE

200 g Salmon Fillet (no skin)
150 g Frozen Green Veggies
200 g Oven-Baked Straight Cut Chips
Drink plenty of water.

AVERAGE SUSIE WEEKS FIVE TO EIGHT: TRAINING PROGRAMS

At this point, you should feel better and stronger as we've laid down a foundation to continually build on. This stage is also when people start to struggle. If you can make it through this phase, momentum will be on your side, and you will be on the home stretch. Stay strong, and don't stop.

At this stage, as we move to more advanced strength-training exercises, the program requires more equipment or joining a gym. If you can't afford extra equipment (it's a good investment!) or you're not interested in joining a gym, you can repeat the first phase's program again, but your end results might not be as good as you had hoped for.

Complete the programs in a circuit manner, and repeat for three sets. Below is the week outlined for you, but if you'd like to swap days, go for it.

Monday: Program 1
Tuesday: Long Walk or Run (more than 30 minutes)
Wednesday: Program 2
Thursday: Program 3
Friday: Complete Rest Day
Saturday: Repeat Program 1, 2, or 3
Sunday: Long Walk or Run (more than 30 minutes)

AVERAGE SUSIE WEEKS FIVE TO EIGHT: PROGRAM 1

EXERCISE	SETS	REPS	WEIGHT
BB Olympic Squats	1	10 to 15	Medium
	2	10 to 15	Medium
	3	10 to 15	Medium
DB Weighted Walking Lunge	1	10 to 15	Light to Medium
	2	10 to 15	Light to Medium
	3	10 to 15	Light to Medium
Sumo BB/ KB Dead Lift	1	10 to 15	Medium
	2	10 to 15	Medium
	3	10 to 15	Medium
BB Weighted Glute Bridge Raise	1	10 to 15	Light
	2	10 to 15	Light
	3	10 to 15	Light
DB Weighted Step-Ups	1	10 to 15	Light
	2	10 to 15	Light
	3	10 to 15	Light
Wall Squat Hold	1	30 s to 60 s	N/A
	2	30 s to 60 s	
	3	30 s to 60 s	
Rest (90 s)			

AVERAGE SUSIE WEEKS FIVE TO EIGHT: PROGRAM 2

EXERCISE	SETS	REPS	WEIGHT
DB Chest Press	1	10 to 15	Medium
	2	10 to 15	Medium
	3	10 to 15	Medium
Horizontal Bar Pull-Ups	1	10 to 15	N/A
	2	10 to 15	N/A
	3	10 to 15	N/A
DB Shoulder Press	1	10 to 15	Light to Medium
	2	10 to 15	Light to Medium
	3	10 to 15	Light to Medium
Seated Row	1	10 to 15	Medium
	2	10 to 15	Medium
	3	10 to 15	Medium
DB 1 Arm Row to Tricep Kickback	1	10 to 15	Light to Medium
	2	10 to 15	Light to Medium
	3	10 to 15	Light to Medium
BB Bicep Curl	1	10 to 15	Light to Medium
	2	10 to 15	Light to Medium
	3	10 to 15	Light to Medium
Rest (90 s)			

AVERAGE SUSIE WEEKS FIVE TO EIGHT: PROGRAM 3

EXERCISE	SETS	REPS	WEIGHT
Scissor Kicks	1	10 to 15	N/A
	2	10 to 15	N/A
	3	10 to 15	N/A
V-Snaps	1	10 to 15	N/A
	2	10 to 15	N/A
	3	10 to 15	N/A
Mountain Climber	1	10 to 15	N/A
	2	10 to 15	N/A
	3	10 to 15	N/A
Side Bridge Raise	1	10 to 15	N/A
	2	10 to 15	N/A
	3	10 to 15	N/A
Side Crunch	1	10 to 15	N/A
	2	10 to 15	N/A
	3	10 to 15	N/A
Plank Hold	1	30 s to 60 s	N/A
	2	30 s to 60 s	N/A
	3	30 s to 60 s	N/A
Rest (90 s)			

AVERAGE SUSIE WEEKS NINE TO TWELVE: MOVEMENT PHASE

You should now be enjoying the fruits of your hard work as you've made it through the toughest hurdles. I am not saying that there won't be hard times, but in my experience with working with clients, working through weeks five to eight is the most challenging.

This is the stage where exercise needs to be an integral part of your life. If you want to continue living a happier, healthier, and longer life, we need to make sure you are building lean muscle mass throughout your entire body.

AVERAGE SUSIE WEEKS NINE TO TWELVE MEAL PLAN

MONDAY

Calories: 1200 kcal to 1400 kcal
Protein: 115 g to 135 g
Carbs: 120 g to 125 g
Fats: 30 g to 40 g

MEAL ONE

Salad Items of Choice: Spinach, Tomato, Grated Carrot, Sliced Beetroot, Cucumber, Spanish Onion
25 g Feta
3 x Small Tins of Tuna in Spring Water
or
180 g Skin-Off Chicken Breast (oven baked)
or
180 g Lean-Beef Stir-Fry Strips (minimal oil used to cook)
Salt, Pepper, and Fresh Lemon Juice for Seasoning

MEAL TWO

250 g Punnet Strawberries

Banana

MEAL THREE

Homemade Chicken Parmigiana:

2 x 75 g Chicken Breasts (skin removed)

15 g Tomato Paste (per chicken breast)

30 g Shaved Lean Leg Ham (per chicken breast)

40 g Sliced Tomato (per chicken breast)

25 g Light Tasty Shredded Cheese (per chicken breast)

200 g Roast Potato

0.5 tbsp Olive Oil (coat potato)

150 g Frozen Green Vegetables

MEAL FOUR

1 x Mint Skinny Cow Ice Cream Cookie

   or

110 g Weis Sorbet (passionfruit, summer berries, or lemon flavour)

Drink plenty of water.

TUESDAY

Calories: 1200 kcal to 1400 kcal

Protein: 115 g to 135g

Carbs: 120 g to 125 g

Fats: 30 g to 40 g

MEAL ONE

Salad Items of Choice: Spinach, Tomato, Grated Carrot, Sliced Beetroot, Cucumber, Spanish Onion

25 g Feta

3 x Small Tins of Tuna in Spring Water

or

180 g Skin-Off Chicken Breast (oven baked)

or

180 g Lean-Beef Stir-Fry Strips (minimal oil used to cook)

Salt, Pepper, and Fresh Lemon Juice for Seasoning

MEAL TWO

1 x Orange

1 x Apple

MEAL THREE

Beef Stir-Fry:

200 g Lean-Beef Stir-Fry Strips

1 tbsp Olive Oil

Vegetables to Add: Carrots, Red Capsicum, Broccoli
Florets, Snow Peas

50 g Vermicelli Noodles

2 x Whole Scrambled Eggs

Drink plenty of water.

WEDNESDAY

Calories: 1200 kcal to 1400 kcal

Protein: 115 g to 135g

Carbs: 120 g to 125 g

Fats: 30 g to 40 g

MEAL ONE

Salad Items of Choice: Spinach, Tomato, Grated Carrot,
Sliced Beetroot, Cucumber, Spanish Onion

25 g Feta

3 x Small Tins of Tuna in Spring Water

or

180 g Skin-Off Chicken Breast (oven baked)

or

180 g Lean-Beef Stir-Fry Strips (minimal oil used to
cook)

Salt, Pepper, and Fresh Lemon Juice for Seasoning

MEAL TWO

2 x Big Slices Watermelon

1 x Apple

1 x Cookies-and-Cream Quest Bar

MEAL THREE

Soft-Shell Taco Wraps:

2 x Soft Taco Shell Wraps

Make Taco Mince from Phase 1

Add Salad Items of Choice: Lettuce, Tomato, Cucumber, Carrot, Corn

Small Sprinkle Light Tasty Cheese

MEAL FOUR

1 x Mint Skinny Cow Ice Cream Cookie

or

110 g Weis Sorbet (passionfruit, summer berries, or lemon flavour)

Drink plenty of water.

THURSDAY

Calories: 1200 kcal to 1400 kcal

Protein: 115 g to 135g

Carbs: 120 g to 125 g

Fats: 30 g to 40 g

MEAL ONE

Salad Items of Choice: Spinach, Tomato, Grated Carrot,
Sliced Beetroot, Cucumber, Spanish Onion
25 g Feta
3 x Small Tins of Tuna in Spring Water
   or
180 g Skin-Off Chicken Breast (oven baked)
   or
180 g Lean-Beef Stir-Fry Strips (minimal oil used to
cook)
Salt, Pepper, and Fresh Lemon Juice for Seasoning

MEAL TWO

Protein Shake:
1 x Banana
250 ml No-Fat Milk
30 g Scoop of Favourite-Flavour Protein Powder

MEAL THREE

Fish and Chips
200 g Baked/Grilled White Fish (Whiting, Haddock,
Cod)

200 g Oven-Baked Straight Cut Chips
150 g Frozen Green Vegetables
Drink plenty of water.

FRIDAY

Calories: 1200 kcal to 1400 kcal
Protein: 115 g to 135g
Carbs: 120 g to 125 g
Fats: 30 g to 40 g

MEAL ONE

Salad Items of Choice: Spinach, Tomato, Grated Carrot,
Sliced Beetroot, Cucumber, Spanish Onion
25 g Feta
3 x Small Tins of Tuna in Spring Water
   or
180 g Skin-Off Chicken Breast (oven baked)
   or
180 g Lean-Beef Stir-Fry Strips (minimal oil used to
cook)
Salt, Pepper, and Fresh Lemon Juice for Seasoning

MEAL TWO

250 g Punnet of Strawberries

MEAL THREE

Basil Pesto and Chicken Pasta

200 g Chicken Breast (remove skin)

45 ml Basil Pesto

100 g Mushrooms

40 g Sundried Tomato

150 g Rigatoni Pasta

Drink plenty of water.

SATURDAY

Calories: 1200 kcal to 1400 kcal

Protein: 115 g to 135 g

Carbs: 120 g to 125 g

Fats: 30 g to 40 g

MEAL ONE

Salad Items of Choice: Spinach, Tomato, Grated Carrot, Sliced Beetroot, Cucumber, Spanish Onion

25 g Feta

3 x Small Tins of Tuna in Spring Water

    or

180 g Skin-Off Chicken Breast (oven baked)

    or

180 g Lean-Beef Stir-Fry Strips (minimal oil used to cook)

Salt, Pepper, and Fresh Lemon Juice for Seasoning

MEAL TWO

2 x Big Slices Watermelon
1 x Pear

MEAL THREE

Homemade Chow Mein:
200 g 98% Lean-Beef Mince
1/2 Brown Onion
1 x Garlic Clove
50 g Grated Carrot
85 g Baby Pak Choy
50 g Frozen Peas
1/2 Cup Egg Noodles
1 tbsp Soya Sauce
50 ml Oyster Sauce
Drink plenty of water.

SUNDAY

Calories: 1200 kcal to 1400 kcal
Protein: 115 g to 135g
Carbs: 120 g to 125 g
Fats: 30 g to 40 g

MEAL ONE

Salad Items of Choice: Spinach, Tomato, Grated Carrot,
Sliced Beetroot, Cucumber, Spanish Onion
25 g Feta
3 x Small Tins of Tuna in Spring Water
   or
180 g Skin-Off Chicken Breast (oven baked)
   or
180 g Lean-Beef Stir-Fry Strips (minimal oil used to
cook)
Salt, Pepper, and Fresh Lemon Juice for Seasoning

MEAL TWO

1 x Apple
1 x Banana

MEAL THREE

Homemade Frittata (makes 6; have 2 servings)
1 x Diced Onion
1–2 x Minced Garlic Cloves
1 x Diced Red Capsicum
1–2 x Diced Leeks
1–2 Cups Leftover Mince Beef from Tacos (from earlier
this week)
6–8 Large Eggs (to cover ingredients)

1/2 Cup Light Tasty Cheese

MEAL FOUR

1 x Mint Skinny Cow Ice Cream Cookie
   or
110 g Weis Sorbet (passionfruit, summer berries, or lemon flavour)
Drink plenty of water.

AVERAGE SUSIE WEEKS NINE TO TWELVE: TRAINING PROGRAMS

You have been going strong for eight weeks and should have seen some great results by now. People probably have noticed the change in your mood, behavior, and appearance, and you should be extremely proud of how far you come (especially since most people don't get to this stage). Your nutrition should be on point by now, so this next phase is all about movement as we step up the exercise programs so you can begin shaping your body the way you want.

The next phase won't be easy, so if you have not been following my routine up until now, I would advise you to remain in the previous phase until you have caught up. This next phase will push your body to build strength and lean muscle, helping to ensure that when this program is finished, you have an extremely active metabolism that will make sustaining the results you achieved in these sixteen weeks that much easier for the decades to come.

Please be sure to follow this training program carefully, and try not to alter it, as I wrote it to ensure you are getting the most out of each session and then allowing adequate time for recovery.

Monday: Program 1
Tuesday: Program 2
Wednesday: Long Walk or Run (more than 45 minutes)
Thursday: Program 3
Friday: Complete Rest Day
Saturday: Repeat Program 1, 2, 3
Sunday: Long Walk or Run (more than 45 minutes)

AVERAGE SUSIE WEEKS NINE TO TWELVE: PROGRAM 1

EXERCISE	SETS	REPS	WEIGHT
Sumo Squat	1	4 to 6	Heavy
(2 min Rest)	2	4 to 6	Heavy
Do #1 Abb During Rest	3	4 to 6	Heavy
DB Bulgarian Lunge	1	6 to 10	Medium to Heavy
(2 min Rest)	2	6 to 10	Medium to Heavy
Do #2 Abb During Rest	3	6 to 10	Medium to Heavy
Seated DB Shoulder Press	1	6 to 10	Medium
(2 min Rest)	2	6 to 10	Medium
Do #3 Abb During Rest	3	6 to 10	Medium
DB Lateral Raises	1	15	Light to Medium
(30 s Rest)	2	12	Light to Medium
	3	10	Light to Medium
1. Lying Leg Raise	3	1 min	N/A
2. Plank Hold	3	1 min	N/A
3. Hip Bridge Hold	3	1 min	N/A

AVERAGE SUSIE WEEKS NINE TO TWELVE: PROGRAM 2

EXERCISE	SETS	REPS	WEIGHT
Incline BB Chest Press	1	6 to 10	Medium to Heavy
(2 min Rest)	2	6 to 10	Medium to Heavy
Do #1 Abb During Rest	3	6 to 10	Medium to Heavy
Lat Pull Down	1	6 to 10	Medium to Heavy
(2 min Rest)	2	6 to 10	Medium to Heavy
Do #2 Abb During Rest	3	6 to 10	Medium to Heavy
DB Chest Flye	1	10 to 12	Medium
(2 min Rest)	2	10 to 12	Medium
Do #3 Abb During Rest	3	10 to 12	Medium
Seated Row	1	15	Medium
(30 s Rest)	2	12	Medium
	3	10	Medium
1. Elbow to Knee	3	10 to 15	N/A
2. Single V-Snap	3	10 to 15	N/A
3. Dual Leg Raise	3	10 to 15	N/A
Rest (90 s)			

AVERAGE SUSIE WEEKS NINE TO TWELVE: PROGRAM 3

EXERCISE	SETS	REPS	WEIGHT
Goblet Squat	1	10 to 15	Heavy
(2 min Rest)	2	10 to 15	Heavy
Do #1 Abb During Rest	3	10 to 15	Heavy
DB Step-Up	1	10 to 15	Medium
(2 min Rest)	2	10 to 15	Medium
Do #2 Abb During Rest	3	10 to 15	Medium
Alternating DB Bicep Curl	1	10 to 15	Medium
(1 min Rest)	2	10 to 15	Medium
Do #3 Abb During Rest	3	10 to 15	Medium
Rope Tricep Pushdown	1	MAX	Light to Medium
(30 s Rest)	2	MAX	Light to Medium
	3	MAX	Light to Medium
Double Knee Tuck	3	10 to 15	N/A
Side Plank	3	10 to 15	N/A
Prone Hold	3	10 to 15	N/A
Rest (90 s)			

AVERAGE SUSIE WEEKS THIRTEEN TO SIXTEEN: FINISHING PHASE

The end is near! After all that blood, sweat, and tears (well, hopefully no blood, but you know what I mean), you are nearing the finish line.

I liken this stage to running a marathon. When you approach the thirty-five-kilometer mark, you begin to feel a sense of accomplishment and dread at the same time. You pat yourself on the back in awe of only having seven kilometers left to run, but your legs are tired, you begin to cramp up, and all you want to do is sit down. You have two choices: You can sit down and give in to those little voices telling you to stop, or you can figuratively punch them in the face, push through, and make it through to the finish line.

That is where you are now during this stage, at the thirty-five-kilometer mark of a marathon. You have come all this way, and you have done all the hard work, but the finish line has never felt so far. It will hurt, and you will want to give up, but never forget: "The pain of self discipline is *far* less than the pain of self-regret." Keep going! You are almost a later-day eater and one step closer to your goals of living a happier, healthier, and longer life.

You can do this!

At this point, I challenge you to start creating some of your own meal plans that work for you. If you are still struggling with tracking your food and macros, flip back to the previous weeks' meal plans, and repeat them until you get the hang of adding in your own food and meal plans. As always, though, if you need help, please don't hesitate to contact me at anytime.

AVERAGE SUSIE WEEKS THIRTEEN TO SIXTEEN: TRAINING PROGRAMS

When you reach the end of week sixteen, you will officially be a later-day eater! You can hold your head up high since you were able to stick it through until the end. Allow me to be the first to congratulate you on the amazing effort, and I hope you realise how incredible you are!

Just because we are close to the finish doesn't mean we are going to ease up on the training, however—far from it!

During this phase, the training program will remain the same, but the sets, reps, and weights will shift up. I also introduce high-intensity interval training (HIIT) sessions. HIIT training is extremely effective in improving your cardiovascular fitness, overall strength, and endurance.

I have provided you with eight of my all-time favourite HIIT sessions that I have come up with over my time in the fitness industry. I hope you enjoy them as much as I have enjoyed dishing them out to clients over the years. If you find them too easy or you want some extra ones, email me, and I will happily provide you with some more.

The key is to give it all your effort while performing the session. Put your favourite tunes on, put your phone away, and focus for thirty minutes—it's about giving everything you have.

Have fun and good luck!

Monday: Program 1
Tuesday: Program 2
Wednesday: HIIT Program
Thursday: Program 3
Friday: Complete Rest Day
Saturday: HIIT Program
Sunday: Long Walk or Run (more than 45 minutes)

AVERAGE SUSIE WEEKS THIRTEEN TO SIXTEEN: PROGRAM 1

EXERCISE	SETS	REPS	WEIGHT
Sumo Squat	1	6 to 10	Medium to Heavy
(1 min Rest)	2	6 to 10	Medium to Heavy
Do #1 Abb During Rest	3	6 to 10	Medium to Heavy
DB Bulgarian Lunge	1	6 to 10	Medium to Heavy
(1 min Rest)	2	6 to 10	Medium to Heavy
Do #2 Abb During Rest	3	6 to 10	Medium to Heavy
Seated DB Shoulder Press	1	6 to 10	Medium to Heavy
(1 min Rest)	2	6 to 10	Medium to Heavy
Do #3 Abb During Rest	3	6 to 10	Medium to Heavy
DB Lateral Raises	1	15	Medium to Heavy
(30 s Rest)	2	12	Medium to Heavy
	3	10	Medium to Heavy
1. Lying Leg Raise	3	1 min	N/A
2. Plank Hold	3	1 min	N/A
3. Hip Bridge Hold	3	1 min	N/A

AVERAGE SUSIE WEEKS THIRTEEN TO SIXTEEN: PROGRAM 2

EXERCISE	SETS	REPS	WEIGHT
Incline BB Chest Press	1	6 to 10	Medium to Heavy
(1 min Rest)	2	6 to 10	Medium to Heavy
Do #1 Abb During Rest	3	6 to 10	Medium to Heavy
Unassisted or Assisted Chin-Ups	1	6 to 10	Medium to Heavy
(1 min Rest)	2	6 to 10	Medium to Heavy
Do #2 Abb During Rest	3	6 to 10	Medium to Heavy
DB Chest Flye	1	6 to 10	Medium to Heavy
(1 min Rest)	2	6 to 10	Medium to Heavy
Do #3 Abb During Rest	3	6 to 10	Medium to Heavy
Seated Row	1	15	Medium to Heavy
(30 s Rest)	2	12	Medium to Heavy
	3	10	Medium to Heavy
1. Elbow to Knee	3	10 to 15	N/A
2. Single V-Snap	3	10 to 15	N/A
3. Dual Leg Raise	3	10 to 15	N/A

Rest (90 s)

AVERAGE SUSIE WEEKS THIRTEEN TO SIXTEEN: PROGRAM 3

EXERCISE	SETS	REPS	WEIGHT
Goblet Squat	1	6 to 10	Medium to Heavy
(1 min Rest)	2	6 to 10	Medium to Heavy
Do #1 Abb During Rest	3	6 to 10	Medium to Heavy
DB Step-Up	1	6 to 10	Medium to Heavy
(1 min Rest)	2	6 to 10	Medium to Heavy
Do #2 Abb During Rest	3	6 to 10	Medium to Heavy
Alternating DB Bicep Curl	1	6 to 10	Medium to Heavy
(1 min Rest)	2	6 to 10	Medium to Heavy
Do #3 Abb During Rest	3	6 to 10	Medium to Heavy
Rope Tricep Pushdown	1	6 to 10	Medium to Heavy
(30 sec Rest)	2	6 to 10	Medium to Heavy
	3	6 to 10	Medium to Heavy
Double Knee Tuck	3	10 to 15	N/A
Side Plank	3	10 to 15	N/A
Prone Hold	3	10 to 15	N/A
Rest (90 s)			

AVERAGE SUSIE HIIT PROGRAMS

These HIIT programs only take between twenty and thirty minutes to complete and require minimal equipment or setup. Aim to complete the circuit of exercises for twenty minutes nonstop, and only take breaks should you need them, unless the program calls for something specific. Warm up before starting each HIIT session with a slow jog or walk on a treadmill.

As with the previous weeks, be sure to track your workouts and push yourself to beat your previous session each time you try the workout.

THE HISSY FIT

Battle Rope Slams x 20
DB Slams x 20
Mountain Climbers x 20
Burpees x 20

GLUTEUS MAXIMUS MERIDIUS

KB Swings x 20
Sumo Squat Jumps x 20
Jumping Lunges x 20
Jumping Single Leg Glute Bridge Raises x 20

PUSH ME OVER THE TOP

Squat to DB Shoulder Press x 20
KB Clean and Press x 20
MB Throwdowns x 20
DB Side Raises x 20

HO HO HO, MERRY CHRISTMAS

Body Weight Sled Pushes x 20 m
Wall Squat Hold x 1 min

DEAD MAN WALKING

Deadmills x 20 s

Stair Runs or Step Up Running x 1 min

Therra Band Crab Walks 15 Right and 15 Left

THE IRON LADY

BB Chest Press 10, 9, 8, 7, 6, 5, 4, 3, 2, 1 reps

BB Dead Lift 10, 9, 8, 7, 6, 5, 4, 3, 2, 1 reps

Chin-Ups 10, 9, 8, 7, 6, 5, 4, 3, 2, 1 reps

Squats 10, 9, 8, 7, 6, 5, 4, 3, 2, 1 reps

Complete all 4 exercises at 10 reps, then drop a rep and repeat until you get to 0. If you are feeling adventurous, now go from 1 all the way back up to 10.

THE PETROL PUMP

Row 100 m, 200 m, 300 m, 400 m, 500 m, 400 m, 300 m, 200 m, 100 m

DB Farmer Walks (25% to 75% Body Weight Combined DB)

Complete the row as fast as you can. Whatever time it takes you to do the row is the time in which you must perform the DB Farmer Walks.

THE WARRIOR

25 x Assisted or Unassisted Chin-Ups

50 x 25% to 75% Body Weight Dead Lifts

50 x Knee to Waist High Box Jumps

50 x 25% to 75% Body Weight BB Bench Press

50 x 5 to 25 kg BB Shoulder Presses

50 x Hanging Leg Raises

25 x Unassisted Chin-Ups

Perform everything as *fast* as possible.

SIXTEEN-WEEK PROGRAMS

TESTIMONIALS FROM MEN

PAUL, 35

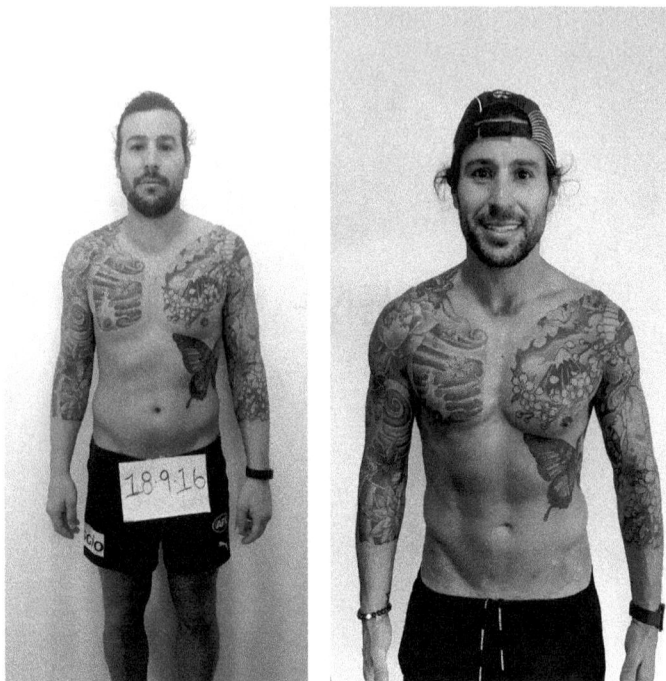

Since starting Adam's Start Late, Stay Light program in September 2016, not only have I lost seven kilograms and seven centimeters around my waist, but I also have a renewed energy for life and training. It has been amazing how different I have felt physically and mentally since starting with Adam. Start Late, Stay Light is super simple to follow and integrates easily into my daily life.

SAM, 24

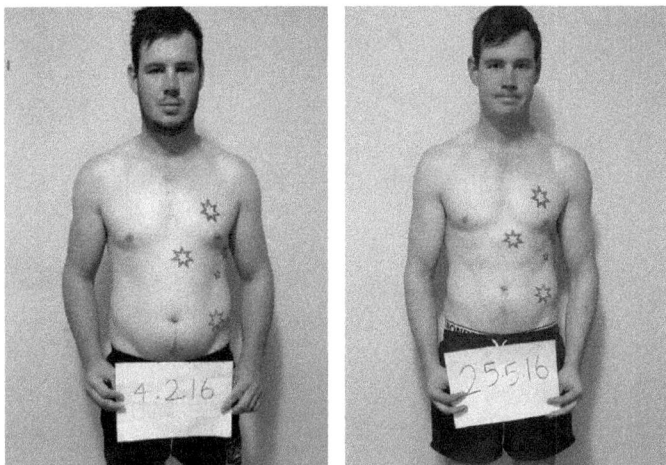

Since starting with Adam on the Start Late, Stay Light program, I have managed to loose the ten kilograms I couldn't seem to get off before. I am now in the best shape I've ever been, both physically and mentally. The best thing about this program is it isn't just a fad diet; it's a lifestyle that is so easy to live with.

DAMIEN, 35

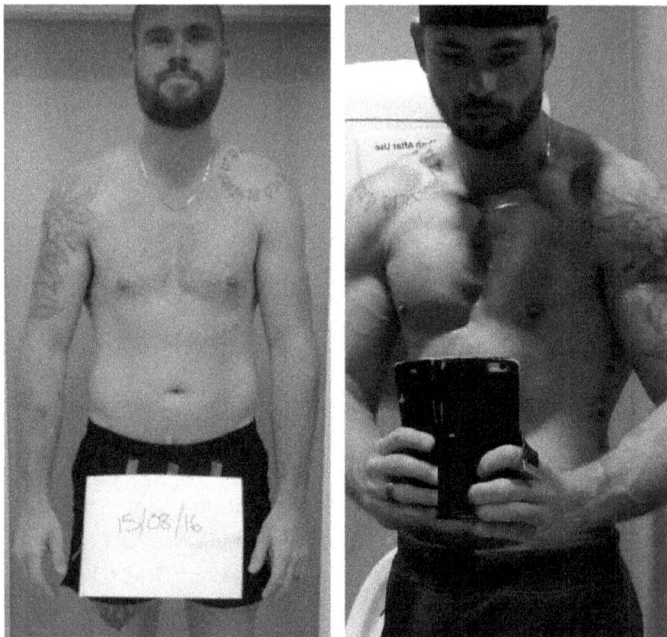

Cutting out the bad habits in my life and changing the way I thought about food has been fundamental to the results I have seen with the Start Late, Stay Light program. Adam has shown me through his extensive knowledge and dedication to his clients that he knows exactly what he is talking about. The Start Late, Stay Light program has not only helped me lose weight but has also given me more energy. The program has also taught me what macronutrients are and shown me how to make different fats, carbohydrates, and proteins fit my daily meal plans. I can now easily calculate everything I put into my body, making sure I only eat the best fats, the best carbohydrates, and good-quality protein. I am extremely excited about my future, being fitter, healthier, and most of all looking better.

SIXTEEN-WEEK PROGRAM FOR AVERAGE BOB

Meet Bob. He's your average man. Perhaps you're like Bob and you sit in an office in front of a desk all day, or you're a contractor, or you travel from week to week because of business. Perhaps you've been looking to lose some weight and build some muscle, and you want to find a way to cook healthy foods, not only for yourself, but also for your family, so you don't have to cook separate meals for everyone. If your numbers fall within Average Bob's range, follow the exercise and food plan in the subsequent pages. If you are outside of these ranges, email me and I will happily give you some suggestions on how you could change this food plan to work for you. These numbers reflect an average height, weight, and body fat percentage for this segment of the population.

Age: 20 to 60
Height: 160 cm to 180 cm
Weight: 80 kg to 100 kg
Body Fat Percentage: 25–40%
Calories: 1500 kcal to 1700 kcal
Protein: 155 g to 170 g
Carbohydrates: 130 g to 155 g
Fats: 40 g to 45 g

Make sure you track your weight and measurements each week to see how your body reacts to the meal plan and the amount of food you are eating. Measure your chest, waist, and hips each week, and write the numbers down. If you're losing a lot of weight and feeling hungry, you might want to add a little more food into your plan. If you're not seeing any results after a few weeks and you followed the program to the letter, then look to reduce the amount of food until you begin to see some results come through.

You may start strength training right from the start in order to build the habit, if you'd like, but it is not 100 percent necessary in these first four weeks. You should, however, engage in some cardiovascular activities. This could be walking during your lunch break, parking further away from your office and walking, or hand-delivering a message to a work colleague across the office instead of sending an email. We'll start heavily incorporating strength training when we reach week five. You'll be lifting two to three times per week and supplementing the other two to three days with activities such as walking, swimming, yoga, Pilates, or cycling.

From weeks nine to twelve, strength training should be an integral part of your weekly routine with two to three sessions combined with one high-intensity interval training (HIIT) session a week. Your usual light cardiovascular activities such as walking, swimming, yoga, Pilates, or cycling should continue to fill in on the days you're not strength training.

Reaching the last phase from weeks thirteen to sixteen, you should have developed a solid routine of exercise, great food, fun, and fitness. By the end of this stage, you should have dropped some weight and centimeters, but more importantly, you should be feeling better about yourself.

Once you complete this stage, congratulations! You are now an official later-day eater and are well on your way to living a happy, healthy, and longer life. Welcome to the later-day eating tribe! The journey isn't over, though. Take what you've learned, and begin to work those skills into the next twenty, thirty, forty, or fifty years of your life. This is a lifelong pursuit and one that will always have its ups and downs, challenging you at every turn. With the skills developed through this program, however, you have the confidence to tackle any obstacle head-on, continuing to see results forever.

Later-day eaters for *life*!

AVERAGE BOB WEEKS ONE TO FOUR: PREPARATION PHASE

The focus during this phase is to develop a routine of not eating in the morning, pushing your first meal until you have achieved a sixteen-hour fasting window and a six- to eight-hour feasting window. I'm not too concerned about what you eat in this stage, since the main focus should be on pushing your first meal to about 1:00 in the afternoon. Although not mandatory (yet), I highly recommend downloading a macro-tracking application on your phone (like MyFitnessPal) and starting to track what you eat in order to familiarise yourself with and learn more about the foods you love.

AVERAGE BOB WEEKS ONE TO FOUR: TRAINING PROGRAMS

As you know, strength training is crucial to your overall success on this program. You must include these workouts into your weekly routine as they will not only help with weight loss, but they will also help to increase your lean muscle mass, which will in turn keep you strong and mobile throughout your journey.

The training program for the first four weeks can be done at home or at a gym and only require a couple of dumbbells (DB) for some of the upper-body exercises. Make sure you track your workouts to ensure you are seeing week-to-week progress and pushing yourself to improve.

With each program, aim to complete the exercises as one big circuit, performing each exercise in the set with no rests. Rest for 90 seconds in between each set.

Follow this program for the first four weeks, but feel free to swap days in order to work with your schedule. Make sure you have adequate time to recover; rest days are as important as training days.

Monday: Program 1
Tuesday: Long Walk or Run (more than 30 minutes)
Wednesday: Rest Day (could do a yoga or Pilates class)
Thursday: Program 2
Friday: Complete Rest Day
Saturday: Program 3
Sunday: Long Walk or Run (more than 30 minutes)

AVERAGE BOB WEEKS ONE TO FOUR: PROGRAM 1

EXERCISE	SETS	REPS	WEIGHT
Squats	1	10 to 15	N/A to Light
	2	10 to 15	N/A to Light
	3	10 to 15	N/A to Light
Stationary Lunge	1	10 to 15	N/A to Light
	2	10 to 15	N/A to Light
	3	10 to 15	N/A to Light
Sumo DB Squat	1	10 to 15	N/A to Light
	2	10 to 15	N/A to Light
	3	10 to 15	N/A to Light
Glute Bridge Raise	1	10 to 15	N/A
	2	10 to 15	N/A
	3	10 to 15	N/A
Step-Ups	1	10 to 15	N/A to Light
	2	10 to 15	N/A to Light
	3	10 to 15	N/A to Light
Wall Squat Hold	1	30s to 60s	N/A
	2	30s to 60s	N/A
	3	30s to 60s	N/A
Rest (90 s)			

AVERAGE BOB WEEKS ONE TO FOUR: PROGRAM 2

EXERCISE	SETS	REPS	WEIGHT
Push-Ups	1	10 to 15	N/A
	2	10 to 15	N/A
	3	10 to 15	N/A
Seated Shoulder Press	1	10 to 15	Light
	2	10 to 15	Light
	3	10 to 15	Light
Dips	1	10 to 15	N/A
	2	10 to 15	N/A
	3	10 to 15	N/A
Seated Bicep Curl	1	10 to 15	Light
	2	10 to 15	Light
	3	10 to 15	Light
Lying DB Pullover	1	10 to 15	Light
	2	10 to 15	Light
	3	10 to 15	Light
DB 1 Arm Row	1	10 to 15	Light
	2	10 to 15	Light
	3	10 to 15	Light
Rest (90 s)			

AVERAGE BOB WEEKS ONE TO FOUR: PROGRAM 3

EXERCISE	SETS	REPS	WEIGHT
Dual Knee Tuck	1	10 to 15	N/A
	2	10 to 15	N/A
	3	10 to 15	N/A
Alternating V-Snap	1	10 to 15	N/A
	2	10 to 15	N/A
	3	10 to 15	N/A
Cycle Legs	1	10 to 15	N/A
	2	10 to 15	N/A
	3	10 to 15	N/A
Toe Touches	1	10 to 15	N/A
	2	10 to 15	N/A
	3	10 to 15	N/A
Russian Twist	1	10 to 15	N/A
	2	10 to 15	N/A
	3	10 to 15	N/A
Plank Hold	1	30s to 60s	N/A
	2	30s to 60s	N/A
	3	30s to 60s	N/A
Rest (90 s)			

AVERAGE BOB WEEKS FIVE TO EIGHT: MOMENTUM PHASE

This is the phase where most people fall off the wagon, so pay close attention to your emotional state and to how your body is feeling, and steer away from stressful situations. Stay the course, and should you have a day where it doesn't go to plan, always remember that you are only one meal or workout away from getting back on track. Don't let one bad meal or one missed workout turn into an entire weekend or week of missed meals and workouts.

AVERAGE BOB WEEKS FIVE TO EIGHT MEAL PLAN

Use the following meal plans for the first four weeks. Feel free to change the days around, should it be easier to prepare the meals in a different order.

MONDAY

Calories: 1500 kcal to 1700 kcal
Protein: 155 g to 170 g
Carbohydrates: 130 g to 155 g
Fats: 40 g to 45 g

MEAL ONE

Salad Items of Choice: Spinach, Tomato, Grated Carrot, Sliced Beetroot, Cucumber, Spanish Onion
220 g Tin of Tuna in Spring Water
  or
200 g Skin-Off Chicken Breast (oven baked)
  or
200 g Lean-Beef Stir-Fry Strips (minimal oil used to cook)
Salt, Pepper, and Fresh Lemon Juice for Seasoning

MEAL TWO

1 x Banana

1 x Pink Lady Apple

MEAL THREE

Pizza: Wholemeal Lite Lebanese/Pita Bread as Base

50 g Tomato Paste

200 g Shaved Lean Leg Ham

50 g Pineapple

50 g Mushrooms

50 g Light Tasty Shredded Cheese

MEAL FOUR

Protein Shake (make sure your protein powder is 75%–80% protein with nominal carbohydrates and fats):

30 g Scoop of Favourite-Flavour Protein Powder

250 ml No-Fat Milk

Drink plenty of water.

TUESDAY

Calories: 1500 kcal to 1700 kcal

Protein: 155 g to 170 g

Carbohydrates: 130 g to 155 g

Fats: 40 g to 45 g

MEAL ONE

Salad Items of Choice: Spinach, Tomato, Grated Carrot, Sliced Beetroot, Cucumber, Spanish Onion

220 g Tin of Tuna in Spring Water

or

200 g Skin-Off Chicken Breast (oven baked)

or

200 g Lean-Beef Stir-Fry Strips (minimal oil used to cook)

Salt, Pepper, and Fresh Lemon Juice for Seasoning

MEAL TWO

150 g Low-Fat Chobani Yoghurt

30 g Protein Powder (mix this into yoghurt)

50 g Whole-Grain Rolled Oats

250 g Punnet of Strawberries

MEAL THREE

2 Lean-Beef Mince Burgers (add favourite herbs and seasonings)

2 Lite Wholemeal Soft Wraps

20 ml Heinz Ketchup per Wrap

Salad Items of Choice: Spinach, Tomato, Grated Carrot, Sliced Beetroot, Cucumber, Spanish Onion (no cheese)

MEAL FOUR

1 x Orange

Drink plenty of water.

WEDNESDAY

Calories: 1500 kcal to 1700 kcal

Protein: 155 g to 170 g

Carbohydrates: 130 g to 155 g

Fats: 40 g to 45 g

MEAL ONE

Salad Items of Choice: Spinach, Tomato, Grated Carrot, Sliced Beetroot, Cucumber, Spanish Onion

220 g Tin of Tuna In Spring Water

or

200 g Skin-Off Chicken Breast (oven baked)

or

200 g Lean-Beef Stir-Fry Strips (minimal oil used to cook)

Salt, Pepper, and Fresh Lemon Juice for Seasoning

MEAL TWO

Protein Shake (make sure your protein powder is 75%–80% protein with nominal carbohydrates and fats):

45 g Scoop of Favourite-Flavour Protein Powder

1 x Banana

80 g Mixed Berries

Water, Ice Blended

MEAL THREE

Peri Peri Chicken and Roast Veggies and Rice:

250 g Peri Peri Skin-Off Chicken Breast Steaks

100 g Sweet Potato

50 g Red Capsicum

30 g Carrots

0.5 tbsp Olive Oil (coat and roast veggies)

250 g Pack of 90-Second Uncle Ben's Rice

Drink plenty of water.

THURSDAY

Calories: 1500 kcal to 1700 kcal

Protein: 155 g to 170 g

Carbohydrates: 130 g to 155 g

Fats: 40 g to 45 g

MEAL ONE

Salad Items of Choice: Spinach, Tomato, Grated Carrot,
Sliced Beetroot, Cucumber, Spanish Onion

220 g Tin of Tuna in Spring Water

or

200 g Skin-Off Chicken Breast (oven baked)

or

200 g Lean-Beef Stir-Fry Strips (minimal oil used to cook)

Salt, Pepper, and Fresh Lemon Juice for Seasoning

MEAL TWO

1 x Orange

1 x Apple

1 x Cookies-and-Cream Quest Bar

MEAL THREE

250 g Porterhouse Steak (cut as much fat off as possible)

150 g Frozen Green Veggies

200 g Oven-Baked Straight Cut Chips

MEAL FOUR

1 x Mint Skinny Cow Ice Cream Cookie

Drink plenty of water.

FRIDAY

Calories: 1500 kcal to 1700 kcal
Protein: 155 g to 170 g
Carbohydrates: 130 g to 155 g
Fats: 40 g to 45 g

MEAL ONE

Salad Items of Choice: Spinach, Tomato, Grated Carrot,
Sliced Beetroot, Cucumber, Spanish Onion
220 g Tin of Tuna in Spring Water
    or
200 g Skin-Off Chicken Breast (oven baked)
    or
200 g Lean-Beef Stir-Fry Strips (minimal oil used to
cook)
Salt, Pepper, and Fresh Lemon Juice for Seasoning

MEAL TWO

1 x Orange
1 x Apple
1 x Cookies-and-Cream Quest Bar

MEAL THREE

Sunday Night Roast:

250 g Free Range Chicken Rotisserie (remove all skin)
150 g Potato (roasted)
150 g Pumpkin (roasted)
1 tbsp of Olive Oil with Salt, Pepper, and Herbs
150 g Frozen Mixed Green Veggies

MEAL FOUR

1 x Mint Skinny Cow Ice Cream Cookie
Drink plenty of water.

SATURDAY

Calories: 1500 kcal to 1700 kcal
Protein: 155 g to 170 g
Carbohydrates: 130 g to 155 g
Fats: 40 g to 45 g

MEAL ONE

Salad Items of Choice: Spinach, Tomato, Grated Carrot,
Sliced Beetroot, Cucumber, Spanish Onion
220 g Tin of Tuna in Spring Water
   or
200 g Skin-Off Chicken Breast (oven baked)
   or

200 g Lean-Beef Stir-Fry Strips (minimal oil used to cook)

Salt, Pepper, and Fresh Lemon Juice for Seasoning

MEAL TWO

Protein Shake (make sure your protein powder is 75%–80% protein with nominal carbohydrates and fats):

45 g Scoop of Favourite-Flavour Protein Powder

1 x Banana

80 g Mixed Berries

250 ml No-Fat Milk

MEAL THREE

Jacket Potato and Taco Mince:

250 g 98% Lean-Beef Mince

350 g Passatta

1 x Small Packet Taco Seasoning Mix

100 g Mushrooms

50 g Corn

250 g Potato (cook in microwave or oven, then pour mince mixture over the potato)

20 g Light Tasty Cheddar Cheese (sprinkle on potato)

Drink plenty of water.

SUNDAY

Calories: 1500 kcal to 1700 kcal
Protein: 155 g to 170 g
Carbohydrates: 130 g to 155 g
Fats: 40 g to 45 g

MEAL ONE

Salad Items of Choice: Spinach, Tomato, Grated Carrot,
Sliced Beetroot, Cucumber, Spanish Onion
220 g Tin of Tuna in Spring Water
    or
200 g Skin-Off Chicken Breast (oven baked)
    or
200 g Lean-Beef Stir-Fry Strips (minimal oil used to
cook)
Salt, Pepper, and Fresh Lemon Juice for Seasoning

MEAL TWO

2 x Slices Wholemeal Bread (toasted, no butter)
1 x Whole Egg (scrambled)
3 x Egg Whites (scrambled)
50 g Avocado
50 g Tomato
50 g Mushrooms

MEAL THREE

200 g Salmon Fillet (no skin)
150 g Frozen Green Veggies
200 g Oven-Baked Straight Cut Chips

MEAL FOUR

1 x Orange
Drink plenty of water.

AVERAGE BOB WEEKS FIVE TO EIGHT: TRAINING PROGRAMS

At this point, you should feel better and stronger as we've laid down a foundation to continually build on. This stage is also when people start to struggle. If you can make it through this phase, momentum will be on your side, and you will be on the home stretch. Stay strong, and don't stop.

At this stage, as we move to more advanced strength-training exercises, the program requires more equipment or joining a gym. If you can't afford extra equipment (it's a good investment!) or you're not interested in joining a gym, you can repeat the first phase's program again, but your end results might not be as good as you had hoped for.

Complete the programs in a circuit manner, and repeat for three sets. Below is the week outlined for you, but if you'd like to swap days, go for it.

Monday: Program 1
Tuesday: Long Walk or Run (more than 30 minutes)
Wednesday: Program 2
Thursday: Program 3
Friday: Complete Rest Day
Saturday: Repeat Program 1, 2 or 3
Sunday: Long Walk or Run (more than 30 minutes)

AVERAGE BOB WEEKS FIVE TO EIGHT: PROGRAM 1

EXERCISE	SETS	REPS	WEIGHT
BB Olympic Squats	1	10 to 15	Medium
	2	10 to 15	Medium
	3	10 to 15	Medium
DB Weighted Walking Lunge	1	10 to 15	Light to Medium
	2	10 to 15	Light to Medium
	3	10 to 15	Light to Medium
Sumo BB/ KB Dead Lift	1	10 to 15	Medium
	2	10 to 15	Medium
	3	10 to 15	Medium
BB Weighted Glute Bridge Raise	1	10 to 15	Light
	2	10 to 15	Light
	3	10 to 15	Light
DB Weighted Step-Ups	1	10 to 15	Light
	2	10 to 15	Light
	3	10 to 15	Light
Wall Squat Hold	1	30 s to 60 s	N/A
	2	30 s to 60 s	
	3	30 s to 60 s	
Rest (90 s)			

AVERAGE BOB WEEKS FIVE TO EIGHT: PROGRAM 2

EXERCISE	SETS	REPS	WEIGHT
DB Chest Press	1	10 to 15	Medium
	2	10 to 15	Medium
	3	10 to 15	Medium
Horizontal Bar Pull-Ups	1	10 to 15	N/A
	2	10 to 15	N/A
	3	10 to 15	N/A
DB Shoulder Press	1	10 to 15	Light to Medium
	2	10 to 15	Light to Medium
	3	10 to 15	Light to Medium
Seated Row	1	10 to 15	Medium
	2	10 to 15	Medium
	3	10 to 15	Medium
DB 1 Arm Row to Tricep Kickback	1	10 to 15	Light to Medium
	2	10 to 15	Light to Medium
	3	10 to 15	Light to Medium
BB Bicep Curl	1	10 to 15	Light to Medium
	2	10 to 15	Light to Medium
	3	10 to 15	Light to Medium
Rest (90 s)			

AVERAGE BOB WEEKS FIVE TO EIGHT: PROGRAM 3

EXERCISE	SETS	REPS	WEIGHT
Scissor Kicks	1	10 to 15	N/A
	2	10 to 15	N/A
	3	10 to 15	N/A
V-Snaps	1	10 to 15	N/A
	2	10 to 15	N/A
	3	10 to 15	N/A
Mountain Climber	1	10 to 15	N/A
	2	10 to 15	N/A
	3	10 to 15	N/A
Side Bridge Raise	1	10 to 15	N/A
	2	10 to 15	N/A
	3	10 to 15	N/A
Side Crunch	1	10 to 15	N/A
	2	10 to 15	N/A
	3	10 to 15	N/A
Plank Hold	1	30 s to 60 s	N/A
	2	30 s to 60 s	N/A
	3	30 s to 60 s	N/A
Rest (90 s)			

AVERAGE BOB WEEKS NINE TO TWELVE: MOVEMENT PHASE

You should now be enjoying the fruits of your hard work as you've made it through the toughest hurdles. I am not saying that there won't be hard times, but in my experience with working with clients, working through weeks five to eight is the most challenging.

This is the stage where exercise needs to be an integral part of your life. If you want to continue living a happier, healthier, and longer life, we need to make sure you are building lean muscle mass throughout your entire body.

AVERAGE BOB WEEKS NINE
TO TWELVE MEAL PLAN
MONDAY

Calories: 1500 kcal to 1700 kcal
Protein: 155 g to 170 g
Carbohydrates: 130 g to 155 g
Fats: 40 g to 45 g

MEAL ONE

Salad Items of Choice: Spinach, Tomato, Grated Carrot,
Sliced Beetroot, Cucumber, Spanish Onion
220 g Tin Tuna in Spring Water
or
200 g Skin-Off Chicken Breast (oven baked)
or
200 g Lean-Beef Stir-Fry Strips (minimal oil used to
cook)
Salt, Pepper, and Fresh Lemon Juice for Seasoning

MEAL TWO

250 g Punnet Strawberries
1 x Banana

MEAL THREE

Homemade Chicken Parmigiana:

2 x 75 g Chicken Breasts (skin removed)

15 g Tomato Paste (per chicken breast)

50 g Shaved Lean Leg Ham (per chicken breast)

40 g Sliced Tomato (per chicken breast)

25 g Light Tasty Shredded Cheese (per chicken breast)

200 g Roast Potato

0.5 tbsp Olive Oil

150 g Frozen Green Vegetables

MEAL FOUR

1 x Mint Skinny Cow Ice Cream Cookie

or

110 g Weis Sorbet (passionfruit, summer berries, or lemon flavour)

Drink plenty of water.

TUESDAY

Calories: 1500 kcal to 1700 kcal

Protein: 155 g to 170 g

Carbohydrates: 130 g to 155 g

Fats: 40 g to 45 g

MEAL ONE

Salad Items of Choice: Spinach, Tomato, Grated Carrot, Sliced Beetroot, Cucumber, Spanish Onion

25 g Feta

220 g Tin Tuna in Spring Water

or

200 g Skin-Off Chicken Breast (oven baked)

or

200 g Lean-Beef Stir-Fry Strips (minimal oil used to cook)

Salt, Pepper, and Fresh Lemon Juice for Seasoning

MEAL TWO

1 x Apple

Protein Shake:

30 g Scoop of Favourite-Flavour Protein Powder

80 g Mixed Berries

250 ml No-Fat Milk

MEAL THREE

Beef Stir-Fry:

200 g Lean-Beef Stir-Fry Strips

1 tbsp Olive Oil

Vegetables to Add: Carrots, Red Capsicum, Broccoli Florets, Snow Peas

50 g Vermicelli Noodles
2 x Whole Scrambled Eggs

MEAL FOUR

1 x Orange
Drink plenty of water.

WEDNESDAY

Calories: 1500 kcal to 1700 kcal
Protein: 155 g to 170 g
Carbohydrates: 130 g to 155 g
Fats: 40 g to 45 g

MEAL ONE

Salad Items of Choice: Spinach, Tomato, Grated Carrot, Sliced Beetroot, Cucumber, Spanish Onion
25 g Feta
220 g Tin Tuna in Spring Water
   or
200 g Skin-Off Chicken Breast (oven baked)
   or
200 g Lean-Beef Stir-Fry Strips (minimal oil used to cook)
Salt, Pepper, and Fresh Lemon Juice for seasoning

MEAL TWO

2 x Big Slices Watermelon
1 x Apple
Cookies-and-Cream Quest Bar

MEAL THREE

Soft-Shell Taco Wraps
3 x Soft Taco Shell Wraps
1 Small Packet Taco Seasoning Mix
Add Salad Items of Choice: Lettuce, Tomato, Cucumber, Carrot, Corn
Small Sprinkle Light Tasty Cheese

MEAL FOUR

1 x Mint Skinny Cow Ice Cream Cookie
or
110 g Weis Sorbet (passionfruit, summer berries, or lemon flavour)
Drink plenty of water.

THURSDAY

Calories: 1500 kcal to 1700 kcal
Protein: 155 g to 170 g
Carbohydrates: 130 g to 155 g

Fats: 40 g to 45 g

MEAL ONE

Salad Items of Choice: Spinach, Tomato, Grated Carrot, Sliced Beetroot, Cucumber, Spanish Onion
25 g Feta
220 g Tin Tuna in Spring Water
    or
200 g Skin-Off Chicken Breast (oven baked)
    or
200 g Lean-Beef Stir-Fry Strips (minimal oil used to cook)
Salt, Pepper, and Fresh Lemon Juice for Seasoning

MEAL TWO

Protein Shake:
45 g Scoop of Favourite-Flavour Protein Powder
1 x Banana
250 ml No-Fat Milk

MEAL THREE

Fish and Chips:
250 g Baked/Grilled White Fish (Whiting, Haddock, Cod)

200 g Oven-Baked Straight Cut Chips
150 g Frozen Green Vegetables

MEAL FOUR

Watermelon (as much as you like)
Drink plenty of water.

FRIDAY

Calories: 1500 kcal to 1700 kcal
Protein: 155 g to 170 g
Carbohydrates: 130 g to 155 g
Fats: 40 g to 45 g

MEAL ONE

Salad Items of Choice: Spinach, Tomato, Grated Carrot,
Sliced Beetroot, Cucumber, Spanish Onion
25 g Feta
220 g Tin Tuna in Spring Water
    or
200 g Skin-Off Chicken Breast (oven baked)
    or
200 g Lean-Beef Stir-Fry Strips (minimal oil used to
cook)
Salt, Pepper, and Fresh Lemon Juice for Seasoning

MEAL TWO

250 g Punnet of Strawberries

MEAL THREE

Basil Pesto and Chicken Pasta
220 g Chicken Breast (remove skin)
45 ml Basil Pesto
100 g Mushrooms
40 g Semi-Sundried Tomato
200 g Rigatoni Pasta
Drink plenty of water.

SATURDAY

Calories: 1500 kcal to 1700 kcal
Protein: 155 g to 170 g
Carbohydrates: 130 g to 155 g
Fats: 40 g to 45 g

MEAL ONE

Salad Items of Choice: Spinach, Tomato, Grated Carrot,
Sliced Beetroot, Cucumber, Spanish Onion
25 g Feta
220 g Tin Tuna in Spring Water
    or

200 g Skin-Off Chicken Breast (oven baked)
or
200 g Lean-Beef Stir-Fry Strips (minimal oil used to cook)
Salt, Pepper, and Fresh Lemon Juice for Seasoning

MEAL TWO

1 x Pear

MEAL THREE

Homemade Chow Mein:
200 g 98% Lean-Beef Mince
1/2 Brown Onion
1 x Garlic Clove
50 g Grated Carrot
85 g Baby Pak Choy
50 g Frozen Peas
1/2 Cup Egg Noodles
1 tbsp Soya Sauce
50 ml Oyster Sauce

MEAL FOUR

150 g Low-Fat Chobani Yoghurt
30 g Protein Powder (mix this into yoghurt)

50 g Whole-Grain Rolled Oats
250 g Punnet of Strawberries
Drink plenty of water.

SUNDAY

Calories: 1500 kcal to 1700 kcal
Protein: 155 g to 170 g
Carbohydrates: 130 g to 155 g
Fats: 40 g to 45 g

MEAL ONE

Salad Items of Choice: Spinach, Tomato, Grated Carrot,
Sliced Beetroot, Cucumber, Spanish Onion
25 g Feta
220 g Tin Tuna in Spring Water
    or
200 g Skin-Off Chicken Breast (oven baked)
    or
200 g Lean-Beef Stir-Fry Strips (minimal oil used to
cook)
Salt, Pepper, and Fresh Lemon Juice for Seasoning

MEAL TWO

Protein Shake:

45 g Scoop of Favourite-Flavour Protein Powder

1 x Banana

250 ml No-Fat Milk

MEAL THREE

Homemade Frittata (makes 6, have 3 servings)

1 x Diced Onion

1–2 Minced Garlic Cloves

1 x Diced Red Capsicum

1–2 x Diced Leeks

1–2 Cups Leftover Mince

6–8 Large Eggs (to cover ingredients)

1/2 Cup Light Tasty Cheese

MEAL FOUR

110 g Weis Sorbet (passionfruit, summer berries, or lemon flavour)

1 x Apple

Drink plenty of water.

AVERAGE BOB WEEKS NINE TO TWELVE: TRAINING PROGRAMS

You have been going strong for eight weeks and should have seen some great results by now. People probably have noticed the change in your mood, behavior, and appearance, and you should be extremely proud of how far you come (especially since most people don't get to this stage). Your nutrition should be on point by now, so this next phase is all about movement as we step up the exercise programs so you can begin shaping your body the way you want.

The next phase won't be easy, so if you have not been

following my routine up until now, I would advise you to remain in the previous phase until you have caught up. This next phase will push your body to build strength and lean muscle, helping to ensure that when this program is finished, you have an extremely active metabolism that will make sustaining the results you achieved in these sixteen weeks that much easier for the decades to come.

Please be sure to follow this training program carefully, and try not to alter it, as I wrote it to ensure you are getting the most out of each session and then allowing adequate time for recovery.

Monday: Program 1
Tuesday: Program 2
Wednesday: Long Walk or Run (more than 45 minutes)
Thursday: Program 3
Friday: Complete Rest Day
Saturday: Repeat Program 1, 2, 3
Sunday: Long Walk or Run (more than 45 minutes)

AVERAGE BOB WEEKS NINE TO TWELVE: PROGRAM 1

EXERCISE	SETS	REPS	WEIGHT
Assisted or Unassisted Chin-Ups	1	4 to 6	Heavy
(2 min Rest)	2	4 to 6	Heavy
Do #1 Abb During Rest	3	4 to 6	Heavy
Seated DB Shoulder Press	1	6 to 10	Medium to Heavy
(2 min Rest)	2	6 to 10	Medium to Heavy
Do #2 Abb During Rest	3	6 to 10	Medium to Heavy
High Bench BB Row	1	6 to 10	Medium
(2 min Rest)	2	6 to 10	Medium
Do #3 Abb During Rest	3	6 to 10	Medium
DB Lateral Raises (30 s Rest)	1	15	Light to Medium
	2	12	Light to Medium
	3	10	Light to Medium
1. Lying Leg Raise	3	1 min	N/A
2. Plank Hold	3	1 min	N/A
3. Hip Bridge Hold	3	1 min	N/A

AVERAGE BOB WEEKS NINE TO TWELVE: PROGRAM 2

EXERCISE	SETS	REPS	WEIGHT
Incline DB Chest Press	1	6 to 10	Medium to Heavy
(2 min Rest)	2	6 to 10	Medium to Heavy
Do #1 Abb During Rest	3	6 to 10	Medium to Heavy
Flat BB Bench Press	1	6 to 10	Medium to Heavy
(2 min Rest)	2	6 to 10	Medium to Heavy
Do #2 Abb During Rest	3	6 to 10	Medium to Heavy
DB French Press	1	10 to 12	Medium
(2 min Rest)	2	10 to 12	Medium
Do #3 Abb During Rest	3	10 to 12	Medium
Rear Delt Flyes	1	15	Medium
(30 s Rest)	2	12	Medium
	3	10	Medium
1. Elbow to Knee	3	10 to 15	N/A
2. Single V-Snap	3	10 to 15	N/A
3. Dual Leg Raise	3	10 to 15	N/A

AVERAGE BOB WEEKS NINE TO TWELVE: PROGRAM 3

EXERCISE	SETS	REPS	WEIGHT
Romanian BB Dead Lift	1	10 to 15	Heavy
(2 min Rest)	2	10 to 15	Heavy
Do #1 Abb During Rest	3	10 to 15	Heavy
BB Bench Step-Up	1	10 to 15	Medium
(2 min Rest)	2	10 to 15	Medium
Do #2 Abb During Rest	3	10 to 15	Medium
Pistol Squats to Floor or Bench	1	10 to 15	Medium
(1 min Rest)	2	10 to 15	Medium
Do #3 Abb During Rest	3	10 to 15	Medium
BB Weighted Glute Bridge Raise	1	MAX	Medium
(1 min Rest)	2	MAX	Medium
Do #4 Abb During Rest	3	MAX	Medium
1. Double Knee Tuck	3	10 to 15	N/A
2. Side Plank	3	10 to 15	N/A
3. Prone Hold	3	10 to 15	N/A
4. Dual Leg Raise	3	10 to 15	N/A

AVERAGE BOB WEEKS THIRTEEN TO SIXTEEN: FINISHING PHASE

The end is near! After all that blood, sweat, and tears (well, hopefully no blood, but you know what I mean), you are nearing the finish line.

I liken this stage to running a marathon. When you approach the thirty-five-kilometer mark, you begin to feel a sense of accomplishment and dread at the same time. You pat yourself on the back in awe of only having seven kilometers left to run, but your legs are tired, you begin to cramp up, and all you want to do is sit down. You have two choices: You can sit down and give in to those little voices telling you to stop, or you can figuratively punch them in the face, push through, and make it through to the finish line.

That is where you are now during this stage, at the thirty-five-kilometer mark of a marathon. You have come all this way, and you have done all the hard work, but the finish line has never felt so far. It will hurt, and you will want to give up, but never forget: "The pain of self discipline is *far* less than the pain of self regret." Keep going! You are almost a later-day eater and one step closer to your goals of living a happier, healthier, and longer life.

You can do this!

At this point, I challenge you to start creating your own meal plans that work for you. If you are still struggling with tracking your food and macros, flip back to the previous weeks' meal plans, and repeat them until you get the hang of adding in your own food and meal plans. As always though, if you need help, please don't hesitate to contact me at anytime.

AVERAGE BOB WEEKS THIRTEEN TO SIXTEEN: TRAINING PROGRAMS

When you reach the end of week sixteen, you will officially be a later-day eater! You can hold your head up high since you were able to stick it through until the end. Allow me to be the first to congratulate you on the amazing effort, and I hope you realise how incredible you are!

Just because we are close to the finish doesn't mean we are going to ease up on the training, however—far from it!

During this phase, the training program will remain the same, but the sets, reps, and weights will shift up. I also introduce high-intensity interval training (HIIT) sessions. HIIT training is extremely effective in improving your cardiovascular fitness, overall strength, and endurance.

I have provided you with eight of my all-time favourite HIIT sessions that I have come up with over my time in the fitness industry. I hope you enjoy them as much as I have enjoyed dishing them out to clients over the years. If you find them too easy or you want some extra ones, email me, and I will happily provide you with some more.

The key is to give it all your effort while performing the session. Put your favourite tunes on, put your phone away, and focus for thirty minutes—it's about giving everything you have.

Have fun and good luck!

Monday: Program 1
Tuesday: Program 2
Wednesday: HIIT Program
Thursday: Program 3
Friday: Complete Rest Day
Saturday: HIIT Program
Sunday: Long Walk or Run (more than 45 minutes)

AVERAGE BOB WEEKS THIRTEEN TO SIXTEEN: PROGRAM 1

EXERCISE	SETS	REPS	WEIGHT
1. BB Incline Chest Press	3	6 to 10	Medium to Heavy
1. DB Front Raise	3	6 to 10	Medium to Heavy
1. DB 90-Degree Side Raise	3	10 to 15	Medium
(Rest 3 mins)			
2. DB Flat Chest Press	3	6 to 10	Medium to Heavy
2. DB Shoulder Press	3	6 to 10	Medium to Heavy
2. V-Snap with DB Flye	3	10 to 15	Light
(Rest 3 mins)			
3. Assisted or Weighted Dips	3	6 to 10	Medium to Heavy
3. Tricep Rope Pushdown	3	8 to 12	Medium to Heavy
3. Diamond Push-Ups	3	MAX	N/A
3. Commando	1	15	N/A
(1 min Rest)			

AVERAGE BOB
WEEKS THIRTEEN TO
SIXTEEN: PROGRAM 2

EXERCISE	SETS	REPS	WEIGHT
1. Unassisted or Weighted Chin-Ups	3	6 to 10	Medium to Heavy
1. T-Bar Row	3	6 to 10	Medium to Heavy
1. DB Bent Over Reverse Flye	3	10 to 15	Medium
(3 min Rest)			
2. High Bench BB Row	3	6 to 10	Medium to Heavy
2. DB 1 Arm Row	3	6 to 10	Medium to Heavy
2. V-Snap with DB Pullover	3	10 to 15	Light to Medium
(3 min Rest)			
3. BB Bicep Curls	3	6 to 10	Medium to Heavy
3. Eccentric DB Bicep Curls	3	6 to 10	Medium to Heavy
3. DB Bicep 21s	3	7/7/7	Light to Medium
3. Plank Hold	3	1 min	N/A
(1 min Rest)			

AVERAGE BOB WEEKS THIRTEEN TO SIXTEEN: PROGRAM 3

EXERCISE	SETS	REPS	WEIGHT
1. Sumo BB Dead Lift	3	6 to 10	Medium to Heavy
1. DB Walking Lunge	3	6 to 10	Medium to Heavy
1. Hamstring Leg Curl	3	10 to 15	Medium
(3 min Rest)			
2. BB Olympic Squat	3	6 to 10	Medium to Heavy
2. DB Step-Ups with Side Raise	3	6 to 10	Medium to Heavy
2. Leg Extension	3	10 to 15	Light to Medium
(3 min Rest)			
Sled Push	3	20 m	Light to Medium
Box Jumps	3	15	Shin to Waist Height
Wall Squat Hold	3	1 min	N/A

AVERAGE BOB HIIT PROGRAMS

These HIIT programs only take between twenty and thirty minutes to complete and require minimal equipment or setup. Aim to complete the circuit of exercises for twenty minutes nonstop, and only take breaks should you need them, unless the program calls for something specific. Warm up before starting each HIIT session with a slow jog or walk on a treadmill.

As with the previous weeks, be sure to track your workouts and push yourself to beat your previous session each time you try the workout.

THE HISSY FIT

Battle Rope Slams x 20
DB Slams x 20
Mountain Climbers x 20
Burpees x 20

GLUTEUS MAXIMUS MERIDIUS

KB Swings x 20
Sumo Squat Jumps x 20
Jumping Lunges x 20
Jumping Single Leg Glute Bridge Raises x 20

PUSH ME OVER THE TOP

Squat to DB Shoulder Press x 20
KB Clean and Press x 20
MB Throwdowns x 20
DB Side Raises x 20

HO HO HO, MERRY CHRISTMAS

Body Weight Sled Pushes x 20 m
Wall Squat Hold x 1 min

DEAD MAN WALKING

Deadmills x 20 s

Stair Runs or Step Up Running x 1 min

Therra Band Crab Walks 15 Right and 15 Left

THE IRON LADY

BB Chest Press 10, 9, 8, 7, 6, 5, 4, 3, 2, 1 reps

BB Dead Lift 10, 9, 8, 7, 6, 5, 4, 3, 2, 1 reps

Chin-Ups 10, 9, 8, 7, 6, 5, 4, 3, 2, 1 reps

Squats 10, 9, 8, 7, 6, 5, 4, 3, 2, 1 reps

Complete all 4 exercises at 10 reps, then drop a rep and repeat until you get to 0. If you are feeling adventurous, now go from 1 all the way back up to 10.

THE PETROL PUMP

Row 100 m, 200 m, 300 m, 400 m, 500 m, 400 m, 300 m, 200 m, 100 m

DB Farmer Walks (25% to 75% Body Weight Combined DB)

Complete the row as fast as you can. Whatever time it takes you to do the row is the time in which you must perform the DB Farmer Walks.

THE WARRIOR

25 x Assisted or Unassisted Chin-Ups

50 x 25% to 75% Body Weight Dead Lifts

50 x Knee to Waist High Box Jumps

50 x 25% to 75% Body Weight BB Bench Press

50 x 5 to 25 kg BB Shoulder Presses

50 x Hanging Leg Raises

25 x Unassisted Chin-Ups

Perform everything as *fast* as possible.

ACKNOWLEDGEMENTS

Mum and Dad: Without you two, I would not be where I am today. Thank you for putting up with me during my childhood years and for always supporting me in my endeavours, no matter how crazy they may have seemed at the time. You taught me that with hard work and a never-ending belief in what I wanted to achieve, I can do anything in life—and for that I will be forever grateful.

Sister: We may have started out as enemies growing up as kids—like any brother and sister do—but watching you throughout your fitness journey and seeing the strength you've had (and still have!) to stick it out and completely trust in the process has been a true inspiration to me. You're the reason I believe we can change the world with this book. Keep up the amazing work!

Clients: I have had the pleasure of working with a variety of clients over the years, many of whom grew to become close friends. It has been a wild journey, and I thank you for giving me the opportunity to be a part of your lives. Thank you for taking the time out of your busy schedules to allow me to boss you around every week.

Amy and Amelia: Lastly, to the two most important people in my life—you make me smile, you make me laugh, you make me cry, and you even frustrate me at times, but most importantly, you make me a better person each and every day. I love you more than words will ever say.

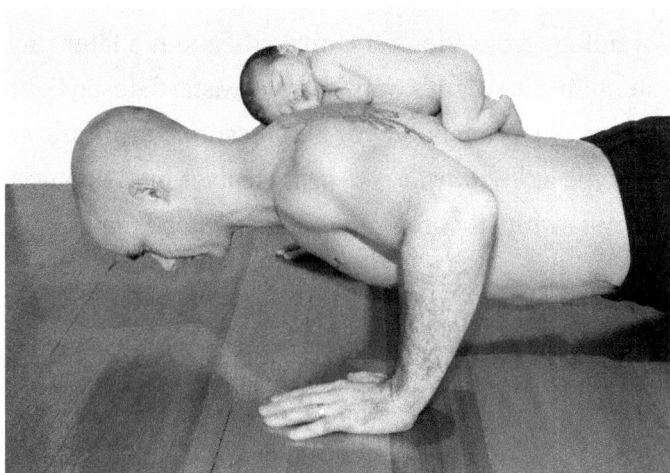

ABOUT THE AUTHOR

ADAM MARTIN is a leading exercise physiologist, exercise rehabilitation specialist, and personal trainer who has helped hundreds, if not thousands, of people live happier and healthier lives—whether that was through losing weight, building strength, or rehabilitating injuries. In 2007, Adam launched TrewExPhys, one of Melbourne's leading exercise physiology clinics. Over the past ten years, Adam has taken his experiences—coupled with his qualifications, education and training—and created a lifestyle that works regardless of your goals, age, or experience. Adam holds a Masters of Applied Science in Exercise

Physiology from Victoria University and is a later-day eater himself. Adam's website is www.startlatestaylight.com and he is available for no pressure consultations on Skype at *live:startlatestaylight* He lives in Melbourne, Australia with his wife, Amy, and daughter Amelia.

www.ingramcontent.com/pod-product-compliance
Lightning Source LLC
Chambersburg PA
CBHW062047270326
41931CB00013B/2976